C0-BJG-862

SHARK HEART

By

K.B. Hill
with
Ava Kaufman

Contents

FOR MY DONOR

Though you have chosen to remain nameless,

To me, your name is Strength.

Thank you for my Life

Together, we live on....

FURTHER DEDICATION

My story is dedicated to the donors, recipients, their families, and the doctors, nurses and therapists who work tirelessly to save their lives. These are their stories, mixed in with mine. There is only so much to tell until the lives of others become intertwined with our own. I carry with me the heart of a stranger, whose family I never met because they chose not to. While I would have loved to have known anything and everything about them, I respect their choices. Maybe somewhere in our deaths, we passed each other, because in my dead dreams, I was gifted the heart of a shark — I never really knew why, until I read the following:

The shark represents strength and aggressiveness when it comes to opportunities and challenges. It forges lasting friendships and works hard to keep the peace. It means you fight for what you want, never back down and have a steely resolve. The shark is observant, perceptive and understanding. And the shark teaches you to enjoy the journey, understand that life has its ups and downs, and take each day as it comes. The Great White Shark has a heart that is considered the heart of an athlete. Its unstoppable beating is encased in a tough, membranous sac.

The shark's heart is safer and tougher than my first heart. And that was exactly what I needed.

FOREWORD

THE ETERNAL WORDS OF ANURAG SAKSENA

A lot of people talk about a heart transplant as surgery. I don't really like that word because it's not just a surgery. It is a transformation of one's life. And what happens in the hospital is a very small component of that transformation. If it takes a village to raise a child, it takes a community to heal a person – an entire community of people to make sure that the transplant is successful.

Ava's Heart is an integral part of the healing process. If you don't have that, you are not going to survive.

Anurag Saksena

PROLOGUE

AVA

Everything was so heavy! I was nailed to whatever was beneath me. My hands and feet didn't move – nothing moved. Was that the weight of it? Was that gravity? There was a light in front of me. The vague familiarity of that light compelled me to move into it – but the weight! I moved forward, but it was not a weightless move. I did not "fly" into this white light – I just had to get there – so I pushed. And the light burst wide open, swirling about me from every direction until I felt as though it was wrapping itself around me.

Someone was there! "Hey!" I called out. But I had no voice.

I stopped struggling.

At first, all I could make out was an outline. There was hair and a body – and wings? They must be wings! The white light fell back. With the weight of my life, chained to my *every single step* forward, I reached for her . . .

Platinum hair fell about her face and tumbled down somewhere behind her. I tried to follow it with my eyes – but my lids were so heavy! Then came a wash of color. Yellow – like the Sun! An amazing yellow dress – everything was so bright. The weight that bound me to the earth began to fall away. The angel smiled at me – her mouth was speaking – but I could not hear – nor did I care what she was saying. I looked for the wings – there MUST be wings! It looked like a flip of the hair . . .

"Ava. It's Tina! Can you see me?"

. . . .

Jesus Christ! Where the FUCK am I?? I opened my mouth to speak – but nothing came out – no sound – no words – nothing.

Voices spilled into the room. I had no idea I was surrounded by those voices – the voices of my friends – the voices of people who had waited for me to wake up. They had waited for me for seven weeks while I slept away a life that had stopped working for me. It was a coma, but God! I needed the rest! Maybe I needed to just give it all over to God – maybe – I just needed to rest for a bit.

And then my whole life rushed back to me – nailing me firmly to the mattress that I was to call home for three more months. I had never really thought about time before, except in the concept of where my next meeting was or where Jade needed to be on that particular day. But suddenly, the concept of time was more important than anything else.

"How long . . . ?" I asked a question, but everyone was talking over me. Again, "how long??" And it was as if I wasn't speaking. That part wasn't a dream. *I had no voice.* I looked back to the angel, standing at the end of my bed. She was smiling – and crying.

"Ava. You've been away for so long . . ."

I was trying to answer her – this angel. But actually, I knew her. She was my friend. She was not an angel – and this – *this* was not heaven.

"Try to stay calm, Ava."

I opened my mouth to speak again, but nothing came out. I tried to get up, but nothing moved. Nothing worked.

Nothing.

But I felt . . . a heartbeat . . .

CHAPTER ONE
AFTER AVA DIED

"I know you were close with Ava . . ." When I first got the call from Milan, I sat silently on the phone. *Were?* I couldn't catch my breath. What was she saying? My chest tightened up, and I was unable to calm myself down. *Stop. Breathe. Inhale. Exhale.* It was as if the person on the other end of the phone was speaking a language I couldn't understand. "Cardiac arrest — Cedars Sinai — That's where we are." I hung up the phone and I told my husband I had to go. On autopilot, I drove, wiping away tears that wouldn't stop flowing down my cheeks. What could have happened? Cardiac arrest? Not Ava!

She's so strong!

The first time I saw Ava, I was training clients at Workout Warehouse and she walked in with Shelby, her trainer. They were identical in many ways: petite, with impossibly perfect bodies and dark hair. They walked in like they owned the world. I always thought that Shelby couldn't stand me. At that moment, all I could think was, "Oh no! Now there are *two* of them!" But Ava was different. She had an inquisitiveness that was captivating. She would watch you and ask questions — like she was genuinely interested in what you had to say. There was nothing insincere about her. Ever. As much as she was like Shelby, she was very different. She had kindness and forgiveness in her, and she understood that things happen and life throws you curveballs . . . right from the very beginning . . .

A ten thousand square foot space in West Hollywood, Workout Warehouse was *the* place to train back in the mid-nineties. Everyone who was anyone was there with their "celebrity trainers" — a term I despised. My husband (who was not my husband at the time) designed and built it from the ground up. Huge, bold, architectural windows with wrought iron panes lined the south-facing wall. Sometimes, in the early mornings when I was training clients, shafts of sunlight would stream through the row of windows, making shiny stripes on the floor and highlighting the tiny floating dust particles that made their way in through the door from the parking lot, which was usually propped open. I loved the dust and light. It reminded me that God was always there. Ethereal, ceiling to floor, light grey drapes blew slightly when a breeze wafted through the room. Industrial lamps that hung from the rafters swayed slightly when an errant breeze floated in. The floor and the walkways to the back of the gym were a collection of uneven bricks and concrete, painted grey to match the walls, curtains, and concrete parking lot outside. The utilitarian carpeting in the locker rooms at the back felt like sandpaper, and there were metal lockers that were probably repurposed from some high school gym. The equipment sat in long rows, with walkways between them, which left plenty of room for a successive line of pirouettes, or round-off back handsprings, or walking lunges. It was a place that seemed like it belonged somewhere else — maybe in Chicago, with a peek-a-boo view of Lake Michigan — but a space like this in the middle of West Hollywood was very cool, to say the least. Michael, the owner, had a deeply sarcastic sense of humor and could be described as Napoleonic. He ruled the Workout Warehouse like it was his kingdom. The clients were the lords and ladies and the trainers were the serfs. Shelby, though, was like one of his queens. She was loud and strong and never — ever — shy. And now, she had a twin.

In addition to personal training I also taught aerobics and other classes at a local studio. Voight Dance and Fitness Center, where studios exploded with pounding music from morning until night, was the place to be a fitness instructor. Since Shelby taught there, Ava was there as well, taking classes. Workout Warehouse and Voight. That was the nineties workout scene in West Hollywood. Everyone was there — actors, musicians, movie and music executives, housewives (that would rival any television show of the same name today), and debutantes. Scripts were read on stair masters and deals were made on the treadmills. While we lunged and jumped and lifted, I was privy to things most private. I was also choreographing fitness videos and teaching my routines to the likes of the Miami Heat cheerleaders and Zsa-Zsa Gabor. When I finished a shoot, it was back to Workout Warehouse. That was all in the early to late nineties. Music was evolving and rap had taken off. Everywhere I taught or trained was changing fast. Aerobics was dying out and personal training was becoming the new thing. Spinning classes were all the rage. I can still hear the music — every song ever written, newly set to a dance beat, intertwined with the screaming riders on their spin bikes . . . it was like a rock/rap concert. It was fun and all had a strange and wonderful feeling of family and belonging. Ava was a force to be reckoned with and, as a client of Shelby's, was a part of the family I was growing to love.

And then, just as suddenly as it had started, it was done.

Every month, there was something newer and better. Trainers were younger with better bodies, and Voight closed its doors. Aerobics had become suddenly unsafe and musicians weren't gearing their songs and beats to dancing or exercising. Then, one night I was waiting outside of Voight for my ride home. A man rode up in an old, beat up car. He asked me if I needed a ride somewhere. I stared at his car wondering, *"Who would ever take a ride from you??"* And I noticed that he was masturbating. I hadn't seen that at first. When I turned to run back inside, the door wouldn't open. I started to cry. To this day, I don't remember my ride pulling up or how I got home. But I remember the locked door.

Strange. Everything about that day was strange. Except for the fact that I knew I wouldn't be there much longer. Life can turn on a dime. A regular day can turn into a strange one and leave you with a feeling or a memory that will never leave your head. And now, as I drove through Los Angeles on the way to the hospital, feeling like I lived thousands of miles from where I was trying to get to, today was turning out to be one of those days.

My mind drifted back to Ava.

Six years had passed since I left Workout Warehouse. I had gotten married and had two kids. My husband and I were running two gyms and spas for a developer in Los Angeles when I got a call from Ava. I was a little scared. Why would she be calling me? She said that Shelby had left the country. Ava had to get her hips replaced and needed a trainer who could get her really strong before the surgery. She had asked Shelby who she should get to train her. "Tina", Shelby had apparently said, to which Ava replied, "But I thought you couldn't stand her?" Shelby said, "I can't. But she is the best trainer. You'll get strong and you won't get hurt." Ava never holds anything back.

"So?" She pushed on. "Can you train me? Where are you working now?" That was in 2003.

And now, it was 2009, and I was on the freeway driving well past the speed limit to get to the hospital. Six more years had passed, and Ava had gone in and out of her hip replacement surgery like it was a blip in her plans for the week. She trained hard to be strong going in, and rehabilitated her hips every day coming out. It seemed like she was back in the gym in a few days. She was ballroom dancing and planning for the next phase of her life as a bionic woman. We started working on a business plan together. We talked about how much fun we'd had at Voight, and why it all came to an end. Our goal was to introduce aerobics to tweens and teens, in an attempt to stop the seemingly new trend toward childhood obesity. Ava set up events in malls and stores like

Lululemon. We invited young kids and taught them aerobics to 80's music and Disney show tunes. They *loved* it!! We had funding in place to get our program off the ground, when the market came crashing down in 2008, and the money offers disappeared. Then, without missing a beat, Ava shifted the program idea to seniors and brought some other players into the plan. I wasn't so much a part of it then. I hadn't seen Ava in a few weeks, when I went to her home one afternoon. The minute I walked in, I knew something was wrong. I was shocked when I saw her. Her body had blown up and there was fungus growing under her fingernails. I spent the next week frantically looking up her symptoms to figure out what it could be. I came up with Cat Scratch Fever. There had been a strange feral cat on her property that she later discovered dead. Cat Scratch Fever is a real thing — not just Ted Nugent's song from the seventies. It doesn't cause what killed Ava, but the feral cat was very odd-looking.

I got off the freeway and was racing through Studio City — down Laurel Canyon Boulevard and over the hill, winding through the streets filled with big, old trees with leaves that hung low over the road, brushing against the roof of my Expedition — my "Armageddon car", as my husband called it. As always, the fuchsia bougainvillea caught my eye as I rushed by. Dark grey clouds hung about Los Angeles, as they often did in February. The depth of color in the green leaves and the fuchsia flowers was so much more intense under a dark sky. I always loved that — but at this moment, it felt more foreboding than beautiful. I felt as though I was pushing the hanging grey out of my way. I thought

15

about everything Ava had been dealing with. Her husband, Michael had been in and out of town for several years, leaving Ava to create a new life for herself, raise their daughter, and deal with their crumbling marriage and eventual sale of their home all on her own. Maybe it was all too much — even for a heart as big as hers.

She had known things were going to have to end with Michael for a while. She had been good with that — but she still wasn't ready to give up the lifestyle that went along with the life they shared. She was going to hang on with everything she could. So God stepped in and took her out of the game.

I thought of Jade. Where was Jade? Ava lived and breathed for her — beautiful and rambunctious and always busy, busy, busy. Jade. Her schedule was more packed than mine, between private school, musical theater, horseback riding competitions and whatever else they could fit in before finally arriving at home every night — with Ava falling into bed and Jade still ready for more. With her golden hair and matching freckles, Jade looked like a character from a children's book — like Pippi Longstocking or Anne of Green Gables. And like her Mom, she was bigger than life — at least to me.

In a trance, I parked the car and ran to the first desk I saw. "Ava Kaufman?!"

"She's in the Saperstein Building."

I moved in the direction they indicated to me, not really knowing where I was going — running desperately to find my friend. I drove by this hospital every day, not ever really thinking of the people inside. I had given birth to both of my kids there. A close friend and client of ours had had a massive heart attack and had stayed there. They had saved his life. Up until that point, my experiences at Cedars Sinai had been new lives and saving another. I could not let my mind imagine that it would be any different for Ava.

I made my way to the waiting room. There was Milan, standing with several other people I didn't know. All were talking in loud whispers. Milan turned toward me. And seeing my bloodshot and swollen eyes, she put her arms around me.

Then she told me the story.

There had been signs that something was terribly wrong with Ava. She was seeing a doctor, but there were no concrete answers. Her little swollen body and fungal fingernails seemed like they should have been a sign of something definite. Farrah, her manicurist, had gone to her home to take her to a doctor's appointment. Through the floor-to-ceiling window, beside the front door of the house she shared with Michael, Farrah watched Ava make her way to the door — down three steps — and collapse on the floor. Farrah was horrified, but the door was locked from the inside and she couldn't open it. She shook it violently, as she screamed to the neighbors. Ava called out to her, "Get David!" And then she went into full cardiac arrest.

David was Ava's dear friend. They had known each other forever, bound in friendship by dance.

Ava met David when they had both been hired to go on a world tour with Gloria Gaynor — the Queen of the Disco in 1975. First, they toured the United States, and it went so well, that they ended up doing a whole European tour. Everyone was in love with David . . . . *Everyone.*

David was a tall, gorgeous Texan whose mother had been a ballet dancer in Germany. Much to the irritation of everyone, David and Ava became the best of friends. Like two peas in a pod. And he would become her neighbor and her confidant. They would sit together on the balcony atop her home in the hills, spending hours talking until the sun had long since set, listening to the sounds of the Sunset Strip coming to life — the sounds of the evening that carried up the hill and dispersed into the night. As time passed by, they appropriately chatted and lived and loved their way into a different life . . . into their fifties. I always felt David was a little aloof. Whenever I was at Ava's house, he would pop his head in the door — see me — and just call out a greeting and leave. Ava used to always say, "If you could just see David dance! He was the most beautiful dancer!" They were soul mates. He painted a picture of her that hangs in her living room to this day. Something about that picture captures the depth of his understanding and tells the story of a true friendship. Dancers are a rare breed. They believe in all things beautiful. They believe there is a dance for all people and all situations. And they believe in the power of the spirit to do all — to heal all — because there is always a way back to the beauty of dance.

David would eventually be the person who pulled her from her locked house that day, saving her life. And what I learned about David the day that Ava died, is that he loved her deeply. I was wrong about him. He was not aloof — just quiet — reserved — because of everything they had already been through.

An ambulance was called . . . and somewhere in her vast house on the side of a hill over Sunset Boulevard, Michael waited through the entire scene, emotionless.

The waiting room . . .

 I looked around the waiting room, and everyone was there. And it dawned on me that no one was with her. I asked if I could see her, but no one was paying attention to me. They were all engrossed in their own conversations. I found it strange that she was somewhere down a nearby hallway, alone in a room. I heard bits and pieces of what people were saying and remember thinking that they were strange conversations. I wandered away, towards her room. I was handed a face mask and a yellow paper gown before I was allowed to enter.

I stood at the door. The lights were very low — almost off. I could see Ava on the bed, covered to her neck with a sheet and hospital blankets. There was a ventilator breathing for her, forcing her chest to rise and fall. It looked so artificial — how her body moved. It was not graceful, but there was immeasurable beauty in the fact that it was keeping her alive. Under the sheet, a square box protruded from her chest. I stared at the shape of it, rising and falling with each forced breath. There was a tube in her mouth and what looked like a thousand bags hooked up behind her head. The nurse in the room explained to me that Ava had an L-vat and an R-vat, keeping each side of her dead heart pumping.

Ava's heart was dead.

I stood motionless as the nurse moved quietly around the room. I felt a lump in my throat and I remember wanting to scream at God.

My feet were nailed to the floor. I could not step forward. I just kept thinking that this couldn't be real. I watched the nurse quietly consumed with the task of keeping my friend alive. Then, as she walked past me to leave, she whispered, "Talk to her. She can hear you."

Tears were filling my eyes again. I could feel that heat that comes with fear and tears, crawling up my back. I don't know if that's shame, abandonment or betrayal. At that moment, I was feeling everything. I moved to her bedside, feeling a heaviness in my legs.

"Ava!" My voice quivered and was barely audible. "Ava, what are you doing here ?" My hand reached for the sheet that covered her. "I know things are tough, but as usual, you are being extreme." I looked at the monitor for any signs of reaction. No change. "Ava, I'm here and I'm going to wait for you to wake up. Okay, Ava? I'm going to wait here." No change. The nurse came back in and told me someone else wanted to enter the room so I would have to leave. I felt foolish. For years, we talked all day, every day, about how we were going to change the world, get rid of childhood obesity, and defeat the depression epidemic by making everyone's endorphins kick in. We talked and talked and talked, and then she would call me first thing in the morning and late at night with more ideas. And now, I had no meaningful words.

I had no words. "I love you . . ." I whispered.

I was quiet in the waiting room, trying to absorb what was happening. Watching all of these friends who I had never met chatting away. They all seemed to know each other. Like a clan. How strange. Ava and I spent almost every day together for two years, and now, as their names emerged in the conversations, I realized that these were people she had spoken of with love and reverence. They all had faces here in this waiting room. These were her friends of twenty and thirty years, whose names came up from time to time. Ava loved her friends. But it had always struck me that she made exceptional allowances for people who didn't necessarily deserve it. And at that moment, in my silent prayers, I tried to drown out the voices I heard, using words like "karma", and "it's not all his fault". I prayed louder. David would later describe the waiting room like this: Raven, a Scientologist, thinking she was going to cure Ava with her "touch assists", Michelle, a converted Buddhist. Mona was a mess in the corner, while Tess stood with them all, chatting incessantly. Then Cathy and Biff burst through the doors, and Cathy called to David, "Oh

my God! David! I'm so happy you are here. I have an audition —
you need to teach me how to walk like a stripper!" So there was
the waiting room, filled with gossip and tears and prayers — and
David teaching Cathy how to walk like a stripper . . . Theater
people.

Ava needed a heart transplant. Someone else was going to have
to lose their life so that she could live. I didn't even know how to
pray for that — pray for the heart — pray for the understanding of
being a donor — pray for Ava — pray, pray, pray. I called an old
client of mine, who was the head of transplant surgery at Cedars
Sinai. He already knew about Ava. Her case was very rare, and
she was not expected to live. There had been some debate as to
whether or not she should be listed, because of the severity of her
illness, and the fact that they had no idea if what had caused the
death of her heart in the first place would kill a new one. "She's
on the list, Tina," he said.

There's a list? Like, who gets into the nightclub and who doesn't?
Ava would never be on a list! She would push her way to the front
of the line and talk the doorman into letting her in.

I went back to the hospital every day at 9 pm when I finished
work. I would read to her or just tell her about my day. When I
would tell her something funny that happened at work, her heart
rate would increase ever so slightly. Sometimes we would watch
TV. I told her about Jade, who was staying with the lovely and
calming Linda. She was cozy and safe and happy. And she was
Ava's reason for fighting so hard. Sometimes I would send Ava

text messages and sign them "coco", like she always did with me when she wasn't wearing her glasses, thinking she was signing "xoxo". Her body was blown up to a size I could hardly recognize. The bed had her weight at 186 pounds. And if she knew that . . . well, let's just say she would not be happy at all! Ava was a steady 108 pounds. A nurse came in one afternoon and remarked about her weight, and Ava's heart rate went up, up, up. I looked at her and said, "Ava! This is no time for vanity. You'll work it off." Even in her coma, she didn't want to hear that she had gained weight.

Sometimes her doctor would come by and talk about her "chances", and I would drive home crying. I remember driving home late at night, utterly exhausted. I got up in the dark and left for work. Then I would leave the gym after dark and drive over to the hospital. The nurses always let me in, and I would just sit there — sometimes talking — sometimes reading — sometimes watching her television shows. She liked *House.* So that's what I would put on. I never really paid attention, though. I was too busy watching the machines — making sure they were working — that they had the correct rhythm of her breathing. I told her about my days and talked about my clients. It seemed okay because it was not like she was going to repeat anything. It was a waiting game of the cruelest sort.

Then the call came. They had a heart for Ava. It was put into her body on her 59th birthday. They say that the day that you get your new heart, is your new birthday. Ava got to keep the same date —

new year. February 21, 2009. It felt like an eternity had passed, but it was ten days.

As I said, Ava was pushed to the front of the line and the bouncer let her into the bar.

Ava didn't wake up after her transplant. She didn't get up and start dancing. They kept her in a coma, and on the ventilator because the disease that had ravaged her heart was still in her body. They inserted a feeding tube. At that point, I thought Ava must be the most carved-up person I knew! She had a mastectomy, a hip replacement, and a new heart. And now they inserted a feeding tube into her torso . . .

But she wasn't done.

It was a Sunday morning. I was wearing a bright yellow sundress. That might not sound relevant, but it is. I drove to Cedars in record time and sprinted through the tower to get to Ava's room. Several of her friends were crowded around the bed, so there was no space left beside her. I stood at the end of the bed, looking directly at her when she opened her eyes. The room was bright with sunlight streaming through the window. I remember the bright light, because I could barely see everyone's faces. Sunlight bounced off of every wall and blinded me, and I was unable to see anything except for Ava's face. It was clear and calm and her eyes were perfectly, beautifully open. She glanced around the room and then her eyes settled on me. I couldn't tell if she understood what was happening or if she was in any pain, but her eyes grew wide, and the slightest smile crept across her lips.

"Hi, Ava!" I said. "Welcome back!" "It's Tina. Do you recognize me? Ava, you've been away for so long!" The smile faded. She looked confused. Eventually, when she was able to speak again, she told me what she was thinking . . . and it was funny.

The next couple of months were challenging. At first, they kept her on a breathing machine. She had been in a coma for so long, that they didn't know if she could breathe on her own. In the end, they had to give her a tracheotomy because she had lost her ability to speak. Ava couldn't walk, talk, or move at all, really. Seeing your friend go from someone who never stops to this was difficult. Watching everything she had to endure was soul crushing. I kept going to the hospital every day. I could not imagine being in her place and being left to fend for myself. With everything that Ava had been through, it seemed that her heart had simply broken. I didn't want her to feel abandoned on top of that. There were days when she looked like she had just had enough. And there were days when she seemed to like this was normal, and she accepted it.

Then came the second wave — as Ava likes to call them. The Karate Boys.

Ava had studied martial arts for some years and she and Michael had become close with her instructor and the men in her class. They helped her get ready for each belt exam. Michael would sometimes go out for a beer with them. It was a healthier time in their relationship — a supportive one — all thanks to the karate boys. Even when Ava had been forced to quit karate because she needed a hip replacement, these were friendships, like so many of her friendships, that were bound in the form of art that made them seem indestructible.

When the karate boys found out about her heart transplant, it was like she had just arrived in the hospital all over again. They descended on the room, and with their encouragement she found a new strength in remembering her martial arts training. It was through this time that Ava found the fight to recover.

Ava's rehabilitation was horrendous. She had to learn to be upright again. They would move her to a therapy table, strap her in, and crank her to an upright position. Her body had lost many of its functions, and she would writhe in pain, tears streaming from her eyes. Eyes that were begging for mercy. Sometimes she would open her mouth like she was screaming and nothing would come out. I felt the nightmare. It was too much, and I will admit that I lost my temper more than once with the staff.

Then Eloka came. He was a physical therapist, sent to Ava's room by some magical force. A man who was truly sent from heaven. He was a runner, and being so, he understood the drive of an athlete like Ava. He looked her straight in the eyes and said, "Ava, I'm not going to hurt you, I promise. And I promise I won't let you fall. I hear you're a dancer. We are going to get you back on your feet."

I remember that day so well. Finally, Ava relaxed. She was starting from scratch, with nothing but her new heart, a tiny, worn-out body, and the spirit of a dancer.

But that was something she knew and could relate to. Spirit.

Eventually, she moved to the therapy floor, where she started three-and-a-half hours of daily therapy, with a very pregnant occupational therapist. They were seated across from each other. The therapist had seen all of Ava's karate buddies, so she pulled out pads for Ava to hit. But Ava could barely lift her arms, so the OT put the pads away and just held up her hands with her palms facing out toward Ava. "Punch here," she told Ava. "Are you sure?" Ava asked. Ava began to punch at her hands. At first, it was just a tap — but then — everything suddenly just came out and she threw the hardest punch she could, sending that pregnant OT clear across the room. "Good muscle memory!" the OT cried. From that day on, Ava knew a full recovery was inside of her and she knew she could get everything back.

Ava was a woman who could fix anything. With everything she had been through, she always came out on top with a positive attitude. Life to her was a difficult dance. You just have to find the rhythms, to move and sway until it falls into place. She had always relied heavily on her body to carry her through difficult times. She had always felt invincible — only now, she could barely move and couldn't even tell anyone what was happening to her. When physical therapists would come by and ask her to wiggle her toes and fingers, I could see her straining and feel her frustration. She had days where she felt like she was losing hope — but she would never admit to that. There were days when she couldn't find that punch and she just had to know it was in there somewhere. She took it one day — one hour — one minute — one exercise at a time, and four months after she died, she left the hospital, going home to a new apartment, a life without Michael in it, and a new heart.

The heart of a shark.

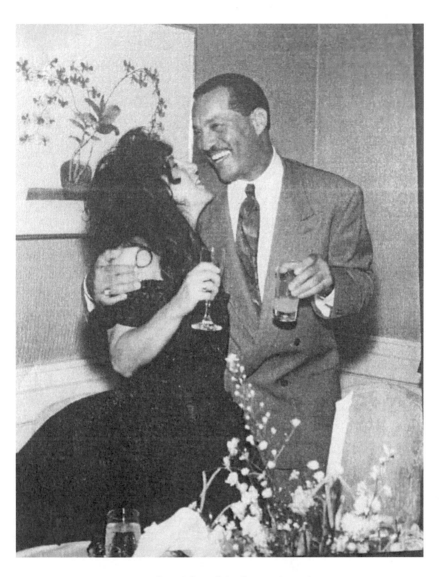

Ava and Michael in happier times

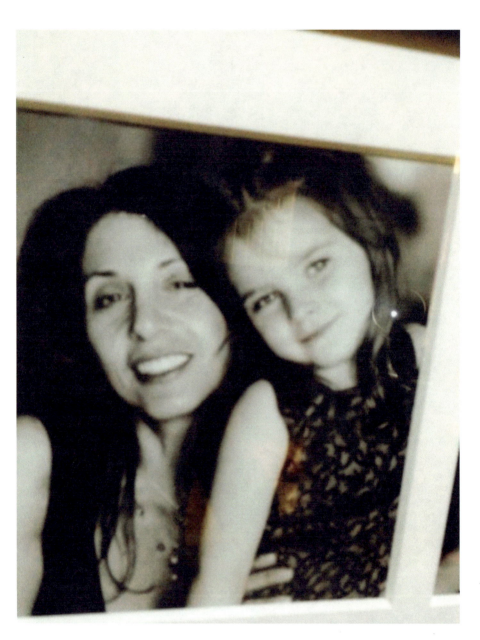

Ava & Jade

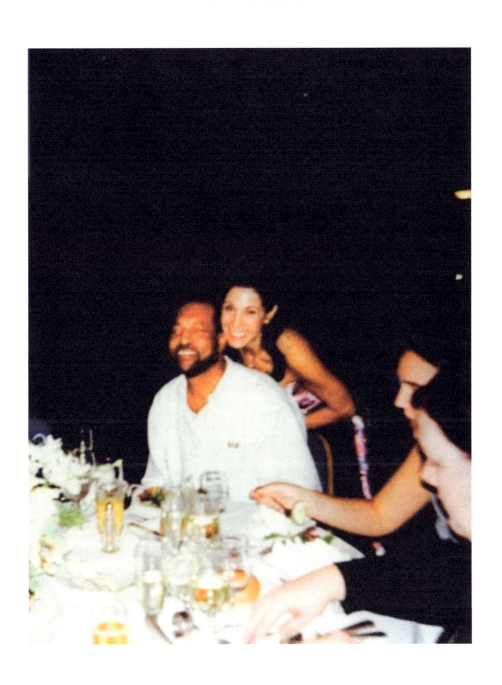

CHAPTER TWO
THE FIRST DAY OF MY LIFE

Ava:

It was my birthday, and it was my birthday. I was 59, and I was zero. Day one. The doctors had removed me from my coma to give me a new heart and told me they had done so. I was still intubated. But I'll tell you what I remember of being dead.

I saw Farrah at the door, and I tried to get to her. Then there was nothing. I slept for a long while, and I was awakened by a brilliant light. It was more of a *feeling* of brightness that was so overwhelming, I just wanted to run to it and be absorbed by it. It was beautiful and had the excitement to it. It was kind and all-knowing, and I just wanted to be in it. Then there was something so familiar. It was a smell — and dare I say not a great one — but I knew it immediately. I grasped for a handful of her hair and plunged my face into it. It was Jade's dirty hair, smelling a little sweaty and a little like the barn. My little girl turned and smiled at me, beckoning me to come to her as the light pulled me in the opposite direction.

My little girl . . . my Jade. I read somewhere that the spiritual meaning of Jade is that it is a stone that protects and supports loving heart energy. I don't think I knew that when I got her, my precious little rock. So, I knew I had to fight. I knew I was going to need a heart, so I told God that if He let me come back and be Jade's mother, I would spend the rest of my life helping other people. But He had to get me a really strong heart.

The surgery happened underwater. I felt my chest being cracked open. It wasn't painful, it was necessary. "Give me the strongest heart you've got!" I could hear the water moving around me and voices talking in the distance. They took the heart of the biggest, strongest shark they could find, and they put it in my chest, and closed me back up. I floated to the surface of the ocean, becoming lighter and lighter as I neared the top. I was traveling toward light and a voice and I opened my eyes. The heart of the shark was heavy out of the water, and the voice came.

"Ava, we gave you a new heart. Fight like hell, Ava."

And I went back to sleep.

So that was death. My daughter's stinky hair, a promise, and a shark's heart.

And then . . . Life.

I opened my eyes again. I felt like I was under the water again, but as my eyes adjusted, I was back in bright light. I looked ahead of me, where a woman with long, flowing blonde — almost white hair — was smiling. She was talking in a soft voice, and I knew she loved me. Her bright yellow dress was shimmering. She was an angel . . . but I couldn't feel anything except heaviness. And I focused on my angel, so I could hear her words.

"Ava, it's Tina. Do you recognize me? We're all here, Ava. Welcome back."

Heaven shot away from me and the heaviness took over. I felt like wet sand on the bottom of the ocean. I couldn't move my head, but as I glanced around the room, I saw faces I'd known for years. They were all talking to me at once. Some were crying. I saw Mona and Barry, Milan, Raven and Tess. Then Linda brought Jade. When she entered the room, I looked at her hair. Dirty, messy and smelly. I wanted to reach out and grab a handful, but when I tried to move, I couldn't.

I couldn't move. Or speak.

It was hard to keep time straight for a while. I would drift off to sleep, and when I awoke, sometimes I would forget that I couldn't move, and it would be that feeling of dread and heaviness all over again. It was six o'clock. Always six o'clock. Sometimes people would come to visit. I lived for visits from people. I needed to know that I mattered somewhere and to someone, but that was a lesson to be learned in time as well. Since being in the coma, I had gotten a divorce from Michael, I'd lost my home, Jade was living with Linda, and I couldn't walk, talk, or even stand up. I was living in a body I didn't recognize for more than one reason. I felt like I was bound to my bed — like I was a part of it and it was a part of me. Why couldn't I divorce the bed like I'd divorced Michael? On the other hand, there was something to be said about not having any control anymore. That was something I wasn't used to. I was a control freak — a real ball-busting boss-lady — but now, I had to let everything go — my house, my marriage, my business. Everything was gone.

Physical therapy was frustrating. I wanted to scream at them that I was a dancer. Didn't they understand? I could do *anything*. Stop asking me to curl my fucking toes!!! Ask me to do a split leap! Or a pirouette.

Oh, to do a pirouette . . . or four . . .

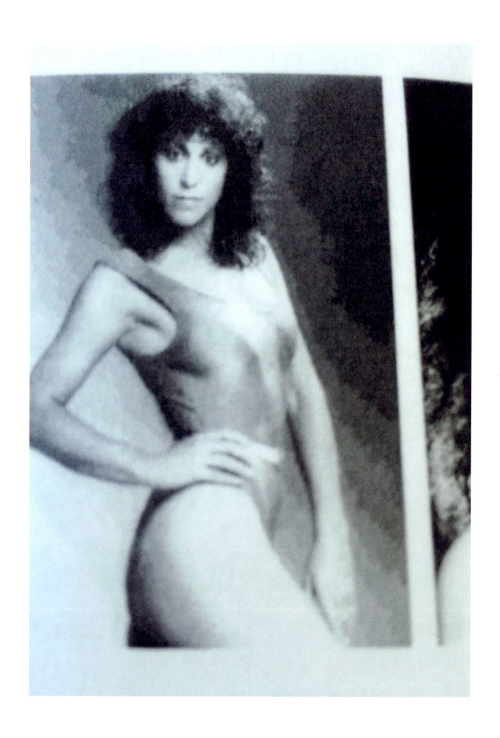

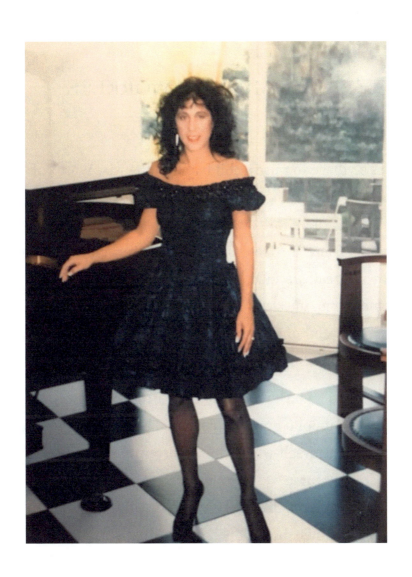

CHAPTER THREE
THE MEDICAL MIRACLE WORKERS

It takes a village to raise a child, and in the wise words of Anurag Saksema, "It takes a community to heal a person". In that community, there are families and friends of donors and recipients. There are doctors and nurses, transplant coordinators, patient advocates and hospital administrators. There are even insurance companies and I have found exceptionally kind people on the other end of the phone when I have had to call them for various reasons.

The professionals who dedicate their lives to helping and saving others are a unique group of people. There are things you must know about yourself with utmost certainty if you want to be in that field. Of course, you have to want to help people. You would need a steady hand. And you have to be willing to spend years in training and then be in debt for a long time paying for that training. You would have to know that blood doesn't bother you or that watching a baby being born doesn't make you faint. You would have to understand that your emotions need to be in check at all times and that you possess the ability to keep others calm when they are experiencing a terrifying moment in their life.

Consider the Hippocratic Oath, as doctors today must state:

I swear to fulfill, to the best of my ability and judgment, this covenant:

I will respect the hard-won scientific gains of those physicians in whose steps I walk and gladly share such knowledge as is mine with those who are to follow.

I will apply, for the benefit of the sick, all measures [that] are required, avoiding those twin traps of overtreatment and therapeutic nihilism.

I will remember that there is an art to medicine as well as science, and that warmth, sympathy, and understanding may outweigh the surgeon's knife or the chemist's drug.

I will not be ashamed to say "I know not," nor will I fail to call in my colleagues when the skills of another are needed for a patient's recovery.

I will respect the privacy of my patients, for their problems are not disclosed to me that the world may know. Most especially must I tread with care in matters of life and death. If it is given to me to save a life, all thanks. But it may also be within my power to take a life; this awesome responsibility must be faced with great humbleness and awareness of my own frailty. Above all, I must not play at God.

I will remember that I do not treat a fever chart, a cancerous growth, but a sick human being, whose illness may affect the person's family and economic stability. My responsibility includes these related problems, if I am to care adequately for the sick.

I will prevent disease whenever I can, for prevention is preferable to cure.

I will remember that I remain a member of society, with special obligations to all my fellow human beings, those sound of mind and body as well as the infirm

If I do not violate this oath, may I enjoy life and art, respected while I live and remember with affection thereafter? May I always act so as to preserve the finest traditions of my calling, and may I long experience the joy of healing those who seek my help.

It's a statement that admonishes to always remember humanity first and to honor the person above all else. And it does not go unnoticed that each of the professionals Ava chose to put in her book, all speak about humanity, the human connection, the value of individual lives and the connection we all share. It's not just through donating and giving the gift of life, though that does create a physical connection between strangers. One that we may not have previously been able to see or understand. The teams of people who brought Ava back to life all had these qualities. And not only the doctors. It was every member of her team. When you realize the magnitude of the community it took to keep Ava alive, you think about what motivates all of these incredible people to do what they do. And what connects them so perfectly as they work together to save a precious life. And they do it over and over again — at all hours of the day and night. The following chapters introduce a few of these people who have remained with Ava on her journey with Ava's Heart.

CHAPTER FOUR
JENNA RUSH - ANGEL ON EARTH

One of many definitions of the word angel is "a person having qualities generally attributed to an angel, as beauty, purity, or kindliness". That is Jenna Rush. She has long, wavy hair and eyes that overflow with compassion. She was Ava's transplant coordinator at Cedars Sinai. I wanted to know what makes a person want to do this sort of work for a living. Jenna grew up in Islip, Long Island and went to the beach every day. Her father was a plumber, her mother was a homemaker and she is the seventh of eight children. Her parents always spoke in terms of "*When you go to college . . .*" And six of the eight siblings did graduate from college. Of course, Jenna is a nurse. In fact, four of eight siblings in her family are nurses. "I have a sister who is eleven years older than I am. I idolized her. When she talked about her patients, it always moved me. I love caring for people and helping them." It is an exceptional group of people who are going into nursing. They truly want to help people. In today's world of Covid, they stand-in for a family who cannot be there as their loved one leaves this world. They are the last ones to hold our loved one's hand when they pass away, and they are the voices who speak the final, "I love you." Angels. Jenna Rush is that special kind of person. She seemed a little sad when I spoke to her over the computer screen. Even a little standoffish. She has seen things most of us will never have to. "Working from home," she tells me,

"I don't have the same ability to help and connect with patients." She is measured and calm when she speaks, and I wonder how she handles a life at home with a husband and child versus what she deals with in her job. "When I was at Cedars, I was working with pre-transplant patients. It was my job to get them listed. I actually met Ava when she was in her coma, but I believe people can hear you when they are in a coma." She goes on to explain to me that they have to run many tests on patients before a transplant can happen. They have to be healthy enough. They cannot have cancer or another disease that will end their life, because the gift from the donor is so precious. Everything has to be in order. Sometimes the pre-transplant interventions fail, and then they cannot transplant.

"Ava was really sick, but she fought so hard. Even though her heart was gone, everything else was fighting to stay alive." The transplant team met every day at 4:00 p.m. Some of them wanted to do the transplant and some were more cautious. Jenna believes that everyone is entitled to their opinion, but that it is primarily the surgeon who is under the microscope. Dr. Simsir, who did Ava's transplant, was her advocate. I paused here, thinking about a team of people who had never met this woman, Ava Kaufman. She lay in a coma, fighting to get back to her daughter, while her body was kept alive artificially. She had people speaking up for her, because they could feel her tenacity. Those who were the more cautious ones had their reasons for why their opinions were what they were. They are not opinions arrived at without much consideration. Every single person on that team wants the patient to live. "There are a lot of myths out there," Jenna says, "but the truth is, we will *always* fight to save you. Always." Once everything is in order, and a patient gets listed for a transplant, they have to find the perfect match for each patient. "For Ava, we had to find the perfect heart."

And they did.

I do wonder how she does it. Her calm demeanor and her soft, kind eyes. People say a lot with their eyes. I ask her if any of it upsets her. "After twenty years, you learn how to make compartments. You put things away. And sometimes something will happen that makes me pause because it is so sad, and I have to remind myself to just breathe."

She lives in a place of constant gratitude. She understands the importance of the emotional needs of the patients and that some cases are tougher than others. Before she left Cedars to work at USC, she worked with post-lung transplant patients. She says, "Those patients would struggle to take a breath. Can you imagine what that feels like?"

I cannot. Nor can I imagine the life Jenna signed up for when she started this job. She knows not every person will make it. She works somewhere in a place where people sit between life and death, between prayers and reality, waiting for a lifesaving organ. She helps them get to that point, and perhaps helps them afterward. And throughout all of it, she deals with the world of medical insurance, hospital administrations, doctors, patients, families and friends. It is said that there are two sides to every story, but there are far more than two sides to this story. To each story of each person, she deals with. Jenna Rush clears administrative issues, and insurance issues, then calls a patient or their family member and relays with patience and love, what all of the steps they must take are going to be. I think about what her compartments look like. My compartments spill into each other, but her boxes must be clearly marked. She has a deep understanding of both sides of the donor/recipient relationship. "A large percentage of the recipient families want to meet their donor family, because for them, this is a joyous event. They get a second chance. The donor families often do not want to meet the recipient, because they are not in a good place." She explains it without an ounce of judgement and with exceptional compassion for both sides.

Jenna sees donors as a very special group of people. There aren't very many of them. Her kind eyes have seen too many accidents and what happens from drugs. A lot of the donors are drug overdoses. I am surprised by that, because I would have thought that people who died of drug overdoses had ruined all of their organs. "Sometimes the liver is too far gone, but everything else is usually okay. But the thing is, these are peoples' family members. I don't know why they got that way. Why take so many risks? And when you think you've heard it all, something new comes up." But it's the freak accidents that give her the most *pause,* as she puts it. "A teenager who dies suddenly from an asthma attack — that's sad to me. You never know what's in your next breath."

Sometimes when I write about people, they tell me stories about their lives, and I ask questions and try to figure out who they are and what makes them tick. I spiral back through everything they have told me, and try to paint an accurate picture with my words. Jenna had some concerns over not being as present a mother as she wanted to be, but I see her differently. In Jenna Rush, I see an exceptional woman who is as perfect a mother as she is a nurse. While this chapter is about her as the nurse, there is a whole person behind the transplant coordinator or the nurse that her patients never meet. The compartments she makes are lined with love and acceptance of the realities of life and death and how the world works. Sometimes it can be cruel, and sometimes it presents second chances for people, and she is there to help move that along. She became a travel nurse after writing a thesis about Upstate New York transplants and where the donors come from. She met a patient who was a heart transplant recipient, who she later cared for as a nurse. For her, it was a sign that working with organ transplant recipients was where her calling lay. And she knew the signs when she saw them. She was a kid who grew up in the early '90s going to the beach everyday, but she always knew what was expected of her. When the time came, she put away her flip-flops and beach towel, and she took her spot in the medical community with grace and poise. And I will go out on a limb here, and guess one more thing. Somewhere on her body, she has what I call an "angel kiss," from when an angel whispered in her ear on the day she was born, "Welcome to the world, Little One. And welcome to the group!"

Jenna Rush

Transplant Coordinator — Nurse

Community Savior

Angel on Earth

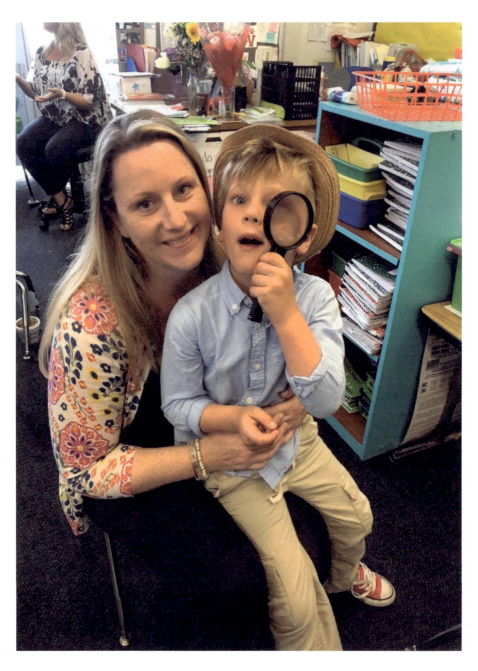

Jenna Rush – Mother and Nurse

CHAPTER FIVE
ALL THINGS QUIET AT NIGHT

I spent a total of two nights "sleeping" in a chair there, at Cedars, while Ava was in a coma. The hospital was quiet at night. It was strange, because when I walked around, there were quite a few people working. They had learned how to do their incredible work, with minimal noise and whispered communication.

Ava was past her coma and her heart transplant surgery, but this was the hard part. She was working like hell to be able to move again — to walk — to dance. But at this moment, her goal was to be able to get to the bathroom and use it by herself. Once she could do that, she could move to the floor where she would get the best possible physical therapy — but right now, she was vulnerable. She weighed 83 pounds and she couldn't talk or walk. So far, she had managed to be able to grasp the rails and pull herself from side to side on her bed.

When I would go to the hospital, I would always ask the nurse's permission to rub Ava's feet. I knew she was in incredible pain when forced into an upright position. I knew that no one had hugged her in so long. I used my old dancer's know-how and rubbed her feet in accordance with reflexology and what I knew dancers like done to their feet. She would feel better. She would know that she was loved and the pain would go away for a short time. The nurses would always say yes, but each and every time, they would remind me to "be sure not to rub above her ankle. She could get a clot." Of course. I was always very careful. Ava was still not really able to speak. But she would smile. With great effort, she would manage to let out a strained "Thank-you" whenever I finished. She was getting stronger. I felt her wiggling her feet a little in my hands. But then one day I came, she didn't want a foot rub. She wasn't feeling well. I sat with her and we watched TV for a while. I asked her a few questions, but she looked tired, so I left.

Over the next couple of weeks, Ava worked harder and harder on speaking and on using the bathroom on her own. Her voice was coming back . . .

Nighttime.

The hallways of the hospital were virtually silent, except for the occasional footsteps of a nurse or a doctor checking in on their patients. A nurse's aide named Fernando came into her room. She was awakened as he drew her curtain back. She smiled at him and mouthed, "Hi."

Fernando whispered to her that he was there to check her for bed sores and move her around. Ava nodded. He rolled her to her side, facing away from him. He pulled her gown apart and rubbed lotion on her back. It felt so cool and soothed her aching skin. Then he moved to the opposite side of the bed, rolled her to her side again, and told her to hold onto the rails, which she did. He rubbed lotion onto her back again, then he moved his hands down her back to her hips and buttocks. He slipped his fingers inside her vagina and moved them around. Ava tried to squeeze, but she couldn't. She tried to scream, but nothing would come out. She was afraid to let go of the bed railing, because she couldn't tell if there was anything behind her.

When he finally finished, he rolled her onto her back, and left her room without a word.

The day after that had happened, Ava was aloof when I came in. She didn't want to be touched — she didn't want the foot rub. My mind back in 2009 didn't go to a place where anyone could have hurt her. I thought she was in a "fuck you and fuck the world — I don't want to do it today" mood. The person I am today has learned that — like children — vulnerable people have that reaction when they have been violated — assaulted — or otherwise victimized.

Each night Ava strained to hear whose footsteps were coming down the hallways. Fernando came back two more times. By the third time, Ava managed to find her voice again. She was able to tell him to get out of her room. Her stress level was growing.

Ava spent the next few days begging to be moved to the physical therapy floor. She was still on the cardiac floor. She felt defenseless. You can't imagine that level of vulnerability, unless you have ever been in that situation.

When Ava did get transferred to the cardiac therapy floor, she finally felt safer. She was so grateful for her heart and for the physical therapy, she feared that if she complained she might be told to leave the hospital. So, she pushed herself harder. She might have felt that getting to a certain point was going to be good enough — but now she decided she wanted it *all* back. Everything.

She was going to dance her way out of that hospital.

Ava finally got out of the hospital in May 2009. She worked hard to figure out what her new normal was going to be. She had to deal with insurance issues and anti-rejection medication. The apartment she had moved into was only for six months, and then she was going to have to find something else. She needed to regain her independence and knew she had to find a way to make a living. It was not lost on Ava now that the company that she and Michael had was called Blue Skys. At first, it meant the sky was the limit! In the end, it meant to fly away to eternity. They had put their money into a beautiful home and a couple of warehouses for their growing business. The problem was that they had allowed help from Ava's Uncle Saul in purchasing the business, and when Ava died, no one knew what any of the arrangements were. Not Michael. Only Ava. She was the one who had been dealing with the business. Saul took everything over, including the warehouses. By the time Ava woke up and had learned to walk and talk again, their home was sold, the warehouses were sold, and someone else was controlling their money. Her home was gone. Her business was gone. And she had been placed on a time restriction for her current living arrangements. Uncle Saul was deciding how long "he was willing to pay for her life" — with her own money.

Little did she know that a fight was still ahead.

Ava set up her doctor's appointments and went to her first one with her Internist. Her doctor, a woman, asked about her emotional health. Ava shared what had happened to her with Fernando. Her doctor assured her that she was going to deal with it, and later told Ava that she had alerted the head nurse of what had happened. Ava said she wanted Fernando to be let go and never be allowed to work with disabled or otherwise vulnerable people — or anyone — ever again. Her doctor felt that was a legitimate demand and promised that she would let Cedars know.

Time passed. It was time for Ava to make good on a promise she had made. She returned to Cedars Sinai to volunteer as an advocate for transplant families — to show them what was possible. She was "the other side". It was her first day. She finished speaking to a family in the waiting room, and was on her way to visit a patient. As she rounded the curve in the hallway, he appeared like a ghost. His long hair flipped back, revealing the face of the man who had assaulted her, as she lay so helplessly in her bed some three years earlier. Her new heart raced, pounding so hard she could feel it in her head. Her eyes locked with his. He stopped dead in his tracks. His eyes dropped toward the floor, and he turned, stepping quickly back in the direction from which he came. Ava's eyes filled with tears. How could he still be working here? He had not been fired, after all. Her breath sped up so fast, that she started to feel dizzy. She grasped the wall to steady herself. A nurse caught her by her arm and asked what was wrong.

With a quivering voice, Ava told her what had happened. To her horror, the nurse informed them that other elderly women had made the same complaint against him. Shockingly, most of their families had called their own mothers, sisters, aunts and friends — delirious and chalked it all up to being sick, old, or on medication.

After everything she had been through, trying to figure out how to navigate this injustice years after the fact was devastating. She had so much love and respect for every single person who had worked with her and helped her throughout her ordeal — so why this incredible hospital had decided *not* to handle this matter was disheartening — to say the least. And he was allowed to continue to work in a place where he could do as he wished because no matter how many women complained, clearly, he knew they were not to be believed. She felt that she had to take action. Ava could not imagine that this man was still assaulting elderly women in the nighttime hallways of this incredible place — and that they had consistently chosen not to take action. She needed to stop it. And she did. Ava hired a lawyer and she sued Cedars Sinai.

Ava told me this story before she decided to sue them.

I chose to include this part of her recovery here because the day that I went to see her when she was struggling to speak and to move, I did not understand why it seemed like she didn't want to see me or anyone else. I realize now that it was the intense fear and panic over these continued violations that propelled her to get off that floor and out of the hospital. It was instrumental in motivating her to get her life and her power back. And I also realize, that this made her not only a transplant survivor, she was also a sexual assault survivor, as well as a cancer survivor – and if there's anything a hospital should *not* do, it is silencing a survivor.

Ava:

So this was going to be my fight. I knew I needed to get back to where I could deal with myself again. I'd made a deal with God and here I was. I didn't know at the time why this was happening, but I knew I needed to listen to everything very carefully. There was always a message, but holy shit! *Why me?? Why this??*

The answer to that has come to me over the next few years. *Why me?* Because I can take it. *And why this?* Because there was a need for it and I knew I was pushy enough — and *am* pushy enough to get as many people the help they need as humanly possible.

I don't like the word, "No."

The shark enters your life to predict and guard you against a harmful person or situation you might find yourself in. The one that means you harm will be scared away by the new confidence this shark energy gives you.

CHAPTER SIX

A PRAYER FOR THE ACHIEVERS

A Prayer for the Achievers

In who we've chosen to be

Things often seem out of reach —

Doubt, pain, suffering, defeat,

Are not the things they teach

So we must believe in who we are,

Keeping Love and Hope alive —

For dreams need dedication,

Determination and drive!

K. B. Hill

CHAPTER SEVEN

DR. FRANCISCO ARABIA - CHANGING HEARTS ALL OVER THE WORLD

Sometimes it's hard to get a story out of someone. You need them to talk — even to brag a bit.

Dr. Arabia doesn't brag — ever — but he is definitely one man who could. He is from Puerto Rico. When he was in high school, he wanted to be an astronomer, but didn't know if there was a future in it, so he went to Tulane and enrolled in engineering. I was a bit curious about what one would do with a degree in astronomy, so I googled "jobs in astronomy". I think my favorite one was a Planetarium Director. I instantly imagined him putting together a Pink Floyd laser show, which was the last planetarium show I saw. I loved the thought of it, but the world needs people like Dr. Arabia to save lives. He could also have attended Georgia Tech, but Tulane had a liberal arts program, so that's where he went. After getting his degree in engineering, he went to medical school at the University of Pennsylvania, then returned to Tulane, working for two years in the trauma center. He went to the National Institute of Health to work in the Heart and Blood Institute, then back to Tulane for three years to study general surgery, followed by cardiac surgery. He then went on to do a two-year fellowship at the University of Arizona. . . . and there's more. This genius of a man sitting in front of me rattles off top schools and institutions as a part of a fantastic journey of a resume. I tell him that his stunning intelligence reminds me of Anurag. "Oh, yes", he says. "Ava introduced us and we have become great friends! We talk about quantum mechanics whenever we get the chance . . ." I don't know if I should say this or not, but I talk to my friends about things like the fact that I have grown two avocado trees from the seeds of avocados that I had made into guacamole. But I digress — because there is more.

So. Much. More.

Francisco returned to Puerto Rico to go into private practice. He had been asked to start a heart program there, but the person who had invited him died before he got there. He became disenchanted, and returned to the University of Arizona, where he started their artificial heart program. He was there for fifteen years, until 2005, and during that time, he got his MBA, which he started at the University of Arizona, and then completed at the Mayo Clinic, after he moved there to run the transplant program. "That was a long drive," he says with a smile. The Mayo Clinic in Phoenix offered him the heart transplant program, which he accepted and successfully ran for seven years. During that time, he got married and had two children, Christina and Francisco (Frankie). He looks a little sad when he brings up his first wife and his kids. "My marriage didn't work out. Too much moving around. It did not survive that." His children are grown and successful. He is now happily married to his second wife, Kathy. She, apparently, instructed him to put a jacket on for our interview, over the shirt he was wearing with airplanes all over it. I like the shirt. It makes me feel a little more at ease with a man of such extreme intellect. He met Kathy at the University of Arizona, but they were both married to other people. The next time they met, they were both going through divorces. He smiles when he talks about her — just a little smile — enough that you know they are a perfect fit.

"I learned something else in Phoenix," he tells me. "I sat at lunch with a colleague there, and he said to me, 'It's good you are here, but what do you intend to be doing in five years?' I wasn't sure what he was getting at because my intention was to move up in the hospital. But he continued, 'You will have to go somewhere else, eventually. To them, you are just a little Hispanic from Southern Arizona.' Looking back now, I see that he was trying to prepare me for how I am viewed in the world — in the United States. In Puerto Rico, I am not a minority."

The other thing he realized looking back, was that this was not the first time he had encountered such racism in the United States. "So I do not use being a minority to get ahead in life, and I have told my kids they are not to use it either." I find it utterly astounding that Francisco would ever need to think about how he was being perceived by the outside world. There should be only reverence for a man who knows and understands so much and who has given a second or third chance at life to so many people.

He remained in Phoenix until 2012, doing more and more artificial hearts, eventually becoming an instructor about artificial hearts. He was offered a job at Cedars Sinai, which he accepted. He and Kathy moved to Los Angeles and she became an ICU nurse at Cedars as well. "Then I had the accident..." He was diagnosed with Acute Cholecystitis, and after putting an artificial heart into a patient, he went straight into surgery to have his gallbladder removed. He also had an emergency appendectomy. However, neither of those was "the accident". In 2017 he slipped in the hallway at Cedars and broke his leg and injured his back. And *that* changed everything. Being the patient was, of course, a different experience. For Francisco, it only added to his vast arsenal of knowledge and understanding of humanity. Instead of focusing on his own discomfort, he used the experience to enrich himself as a doctor and as a teacher. "I understand what it is to be a patient. They have much less power than we do as doctors." He tells me about a patient he had when he was a fellow. "He was waiting for a transplant when he coded. And he coded for twenty minutes. We shocked him one more time. When I left that night, I didn't think he would make it, but when I got back to the hospital the next morning, he was awake and talking. He told me that he had chest pain, then went to a beautiful place with blue light and a tunnel. He told me it made him feel so good. His descriptions were so intense — it was incredible." He said he thinks about that more as he gets older. "I want to have no pain."

I find his humility almost disarming. My questions float through different stages of an extraordinary life. A life that has affected countless people and one in which he has learned about so many incredible things, like how to put a new heart into a person's body.

And he has taught so many like-minded people and saved so many lives. I try to wrap my head around anyone being dismissive or racist toward him. It must be that it makes them uncomfortable to be around someone who is so quietly brilliant. Maybe I am giving those people too much credit. "When I am invited to give a presentation on artificial hearts, people like to challenge me. I think it is primarily because of my accent. I get questioned more than other people, and I had to learn to defend myself. Now, I look forward to it." He speaks triumphantly and with the kind of resolve that comes with a lifetime of studying the most incredible mechanisms on the planet. When he gives a lecture, he plays a clip from the movie, *Ironman*, ending with his favorite line, when Tony Stark asks Pepper Potts, "Can you change my heart?" And that's what he teaches about. It's *The Bionic Man*. It's *Ironman*. I am curious as to whether that means this new artificial heart is limitless when it comes to breathing. "Yes," he says. "But the rest of the body systems are the same as before — so they may not be able to keep up . . . yet!" Quantum mechanics, artificial intelligence and a new heart that is in clinical trials that is virtually silent. He tells me, "I like science fiction and things that are possibilities for humanity someday."

Possibilities for humanity. How many people think like that?

Every single scientific discovery has been based on possibilities. On challenging what we believe are our limits and imagining something better, more fantastic, more magical until it comes to life. That is where Francisco's mind goes. I am fascinated to know what he was like as a little boy, but he just shrugs it off. "I wanted to design cars and airplanes." Of course, he did.

Possibilities.

Our conversation shifts again. I ask him about transference. I want to know, what is the implication of changing someone's heart? "We know that there are genetic changes," he tells me. "The recipient has the genetic material of the donor inside of their body. Does that do anything? You cannot rule it out. It may be psychological, but it may be physical, actual." But really, what is the difference? They all make up the person. Francisco's understanding of the human heart goes far beyond what he learned in medical school. He has spoken to patients and listened to their experiences. He has been a patient himself and understands that these surgeries are life-altering. Changing someone's heart has implications far beyond what we can ever imagine. It's not just surgery. It's a second chance or a new beginning. It's honoring the life of a donor and it is honoring the people who create artificial hearts. It is honoring the patient.

Life.

"Ava . . . Ava needs to be a bigger operation. More people need what she can offer, but she cannot offer what she doesn't have access to."

So, how did he meet Ava? Francisco smiles. She was in the hospital one day when she was still at Cedars. A young woman needed an artificial heart. She was from Texas. No one there wanted to do it. She was Puerto Rican. I knew where she was from and I met her family. Ava was talking to her. She was in her thirties and she had a congenital heart defect. I did her heart transplant a year later, but she only lasted six months."

He takes a moment.

"Humility," he says, "comes from knowing things don't always work."

Dr. Francisco Arabia

Doctor, Teacher, Husband, Father, Grandfather

Humbled by Humanity

Changing Hearts All Over the World

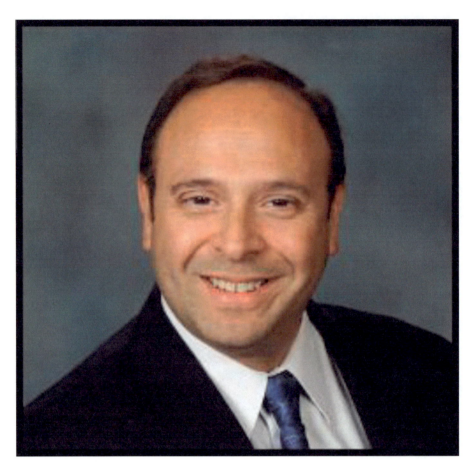

Dr. Francisco Arabia – The Humble Genius

CHAPTER EIGHT
BEFORE

Ava:

I don't want this book to just be about me, but I do think it's important to tell the whole story, and every story has a beginning. There's always a pathway that leads you through your life. I'll admit I (frequently) stepped off that pathway. I couldn't help it. The music made me do it!

Growing up in Yonkers with my family did two things for me: First, it taught me about love. My father loved my mother to the moon and back! And while she mussed and fussed about him needing to make more money, I knew she loved him back. I was the eldest of three kids. When I was four, Mona was born. She was my new little play doll. I absolutely adored her! My brother Barry didn't come along for six more years, so by then, I was old enough to babysit! Mona and I loved him like he was our forever puppy. Just like with Mona, Barry was our little bundle of joy. We played with him, tortured him, loved him, and handed him back to our mother when he had had enough of us. Sometimes, when my mother would get a little fed up with my antics, she would send me to my room. My letters of apology, beginning at the age of six, would be signed, "Sincerely, The Black Hand." When I was in second grade, I took the bus to Gimbles in White Plains, with my friends from up the street. They were twins. We couldn't have been more than seven or eight years old. When I walked into that store, just my twin friends and me, I thought to myself, "You have to remember this moment for the rest of your life." It was absolutely thrilling — being free of any parental control and having a little of my own money to spend however I wanted. Times are different now.

We had a great house on a typical middle class street. There were yards with fresh-cut grass and yards that were not so manicured. My favorite thing about that street was when it rained. I would sit with my father on the porch for hours and watch the thundershowers. And when it was done, I loved the smell of the grass, trees and concrete all mixed together — washed clean for another day. I had two grandmothers — one a typical "Jewish grandmother", with a heavy New York accent who liked to make me eat. People may read that and find some sort of offense in it, but that woman was as strong as she was loving and as crazy as she was brilliant. Most people don't get someone like that in their lives. My other grandmother was the polar opposite. She was a hippy — a retired opera singer who lived on a farm out in the country in Stanfordville. I would spend my summers with her — usually siblingless. She loved lilacs. Her farm was filled with fruit trees and pathways for me to explore. I danced my way through hot, sticky summers with a beautiful old woman, who lived on 69 acres — and when that final summer sun set, and my father came to pick me up, I would wrap my arms around my grandmother, gathering her scent into my soul so that I wouldn't forget her.

I was a combination of my two grandmothers: strong and loving, a little crazy, and a touch of that girl who danced by the light of the moon in her nightgown.

My mother died in 2002 and my father in 2009, shortly after I received my heart transplant. After my mother died, we had all made an agreement to take turns going down to Boca Raton, Florida, to visit my Dad. Just around Christmas in 2008, Jade and I went to visit him. My body hadn't blown up yet, but I was itchy. My father told me, "I have the best itching cream!" (Parents always have the best remedies.) We had a wonderful time there. That was the last time I saw my Dad. I did get to talk to him the night before he died. I told him to "Go be with Mommy." And he did. While, as I said, this story isn't just about me; this is the journey that created my foundation. It's a journey we all have, and mine was born out of love and boredom, strong family ties and broken ones, and lots and lots of ambition. This brings me to the second thing: I realized I wanted something different. It was a happy childhood, but, as lovely as everything was, it was *so* boring! I had to get away as soon as I could, and dancing was going to be my ticket out.

Dance was my escape to a better life — at least in my mind it was. By the time I was twelve years old, I was taking the train into Manhattan to my dance lessons by myself, and at 13, I tried out for the New York City Ballet School, under the direction of George Balanchine. He told me I was too fat and I had bad feet — but really, what did he know? So I went to Metropolitan Ballet, auditioned, and got into their program. Like my Jewish grandmother, I wasn't going to take no for an answer. Mona, on the other hand, was told she, too, had bad feet, so she quit. So while George Ballanchine may have had something to do with the trajectory of Mona's life, he was but a footnote in mine.

Mona and I were as close as two sisters could be. She went to UCSB and met the most gorgeous guy ever. His name was Kevin. They moved back east and got married. She got her master's degree in social work and he went to law school, and I lived right around the corner from them. I was dating a guy named Ken at the time, and the four of us painted the town red! We would go out dancing, partying and laughing our way through Manhattan. I was dancing to my dream and Kevin had decided to take a year off and wait tables while Mona finished her master's degree. Everything was going great. Mona was going to be a social worker, and Kevin was going to be a lawyer. They were madly in love. Then, Mona's life turned abruptly in a way that is not my story to tell. Kevin was gone as suddenly as he had appeared, and she dropped out of social work and got a business degree. She and Kevin divorced, and just like that, another man stepped in — a doctor named Jerry. And as Fate would have it, the very day Jerry asked Mona to marry him, Kevin took his own life.

When I think back on that time, as with many of my life stories, it is like a scene in a play. The stage is filled with people. They are all laughing and there is music and dancing. Suddenly someone walks alone toward the front of the stage. Everyone else has fallen back into the wings, and the music turns sad.

After that, Mona and I were never the same again. I loved my sister so much, but there was a sadness in her that I could not carry with me throughout my life. I used to wonder what it was about some people that made them seem to morph into their spouses. She became more religious than we ever were growing up. Jerry was not fun, and Mona followed in his footsteps. My baby doll was no more. She now saw me as spoiled and unrealistic, whereas I had been creative and fun when we were young. When I danced, she didn't come to watch me and when I called her to talk about my tours or my life, she barely listened.

I needed to go to work, so after majoring in dance at NYU, I got a job working at Capezio. They were great to me there, because I ran the place! I discovered Milliskin with Estelle Sommers, who I called Mrs. Capezio. Milliskin was a four-way stretchy material that fit like a glove. Gone were the gaps in cotton bodysuits and leotards. It was like a second skin! But it only came in black and white . . . so being the creative young woman I was, I would take leotards home and dye them different colors. We fit all of the greatest dancers from the greatest companies. I remembered getting my very first pair of pointe shoes at Capezio, and now the whole store was my oyster. It was a great job and it was fun for a while. I met interesting people and I was making money. I loved it, but I loved dancing more. So just like that, I quit. And my life became about hours and hours in a dance studio, perfecting my technique and becoming a stronger dancer. As soon as I began auditioning, I got my first job dancing as a backup dancer for Gloria Gaynor on her "Disco Queen Tour". I twirled and jumped and danced all over the world with some of the most incredible partners a girl could ever ask for. Every single day excited me and every single night, as the stage lit up, I came alive. During that time, I studied with Fred Benjamin, who was my favorite teacher of all time. My partner in his Saturday morning classes was Ben Harney, who later won a Tony Award for DreamGirls. I also danced with Ron Farella and went to Paris with Jo-Jo Smith's company. This was what I was put on this planet for . . . And then . . . There was Larry Riley. When I think about him today, I feel like no one ever loved anyone like I loved Larry. He was the reason I came to Los Angeles. He had moved out here to open DreamGirls in Los Angeles and shot A Soldier's Story with Denzel Washington and I followed him. But my love wasn't enough to make it work, so after ten years, I moved on. That may sound abrupt, but it was just that. Something works until it doesn't, and you move on.

Who would have thought that the whole point of the endless hours of dance and discipline was all meant for something entirely different? All those years ago, when I would dance through *any* amount of pain for the applause of an audience, who would ever have thought that the day would come when I could no longer do any of that? I could never have imagined the life of a wife and business person, a daughter who was my gift from God and who became my only reason for fighting to live, and that would be the only way I knew to fight my way back to being able to stand, walk, talk . . . and eventually, find my true purpose.

And first, of course, there was Michael. I think that once in everybody's life, they get to at least brush past their one true love. If your heart is open, you feel it when it happens. And my heart was wide open, like the Grand Canyon. Michael was beautiful. I loved Michael with every ounce of my being.

I had moved to Los Angeles to be with my boyfriend — or so I thought. Since Larry and I were done, I was out there on my own. I was at some friend's house. I accidentally walked into a room where Michael was getting a massage. And as I said, Michael was *beautiful*. He asked me if I was going to be at the New Year's Eve party that night. I was. I wore black leather pants and a red sweater. We spent the night together — and that was it. Me and Michael. It's amazing what black leather pants can do.

We were inseparable. I moved out of my tiny apartment and we moved in together.

Michael had a little delivery company called Blue Skys. Together, we grew it into the moving company to the stars. We did the Four Seasons in Beverly Hills, The Regent Beverly Wilshire, and the Four Seasons in Kona and Maui. We went from having nothing to having so much very quickly — something that became beyond my capabilities — or at least that's how I felt at the time. I worked in the office and got us customers. Michael went on every moving job and helped the guys with the labor. It was his company and he was the boss, but his work ethic was that he knew he was never too good to do the heavy lifting. And I guess it was the heavy lifting that did him in. Eventually, he severely injured his back. I think when the thing you have always known you could do — no matter what — is suddenly taken away from you, it can really take you down. He couldn't do the "heavy lifting" anymore — in fact, he couldn't do *any* lifting. His broken back also broke his spirit, and whatever belief he had in himself went with it. Every last morsel of comfort he deserved was stolen from him and he couldn't help but be angry. I don't even know where he is anymore, but when I allow myself to be swept back to that time when we met — that first time when I thought he was the most incredible man I'd ever seen — the times when we would lay wrapped in a passionate embrace — and how we moved seamlessly from a little company to a thriving one — I am aware of two, undeniable things. What we accomplished, we did together, because for a brief moment in time, we were two people, so perfectly suited for each other, we could have done anything and made it perfect. And for an even briefer moment, I had true love.

For people who knew us all along, many thought that Michael was, in the end, a monster. But he wasn't. He was broken, just like I was. Now, there was no one left to comfort him or help him anymore, because they were all gathered around my bed, praying for me to live. But I *had* lived! And I had loved like a fairy tale or like the most incredible love story.

. . . Walking alone to the front of the stage while the music grew sad . . .

When things change — as things do — we have to make decisions on how we want to deal with those changes. I wanted to be a mom. I had wanted to have a family, but I had one miscarriage after another. So we got Jade. For me, Jade was my new greatest love. Being a mom killed my desire to run our business. I just wanted to be with her — every minute I could. Jade and I would go to the barn and I would watch her ride. She was one of those rare kids who just became one with the horse when she got on. She had no fear because they were one and the same. Her hair would be whipping out from beneath her helmet, and her horse's tail would be flying in the exact same way.

During that same time, Michael had a friend named Arthur — an older gentleman who was in real estate. Arthur liked cocaine. They traveled together. They went to Peru and then to Thailand. They got along well and Michael loved traveling to other places. I knew he was with other women, but I had Jade. He was looking for something — always looking outward, never wanting to look inward.

I knew that one day, I would have to come to terms with my marriage, but it was never today. In my heart of hearts, I had the kind of love that most people don't get to have. I would talk about our great sex and our successful business, but deep inside, Michael made my heart soar — every single time he walked through the door. And I felt his love for me just as strongly. Maybe that's the trade-off, when you love so openly and wholly — that when it's done . . . well . . . that's when the first crack rippled through my heart.

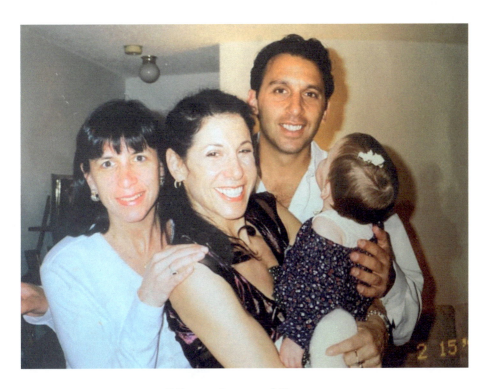

Mona, Ava and Barry

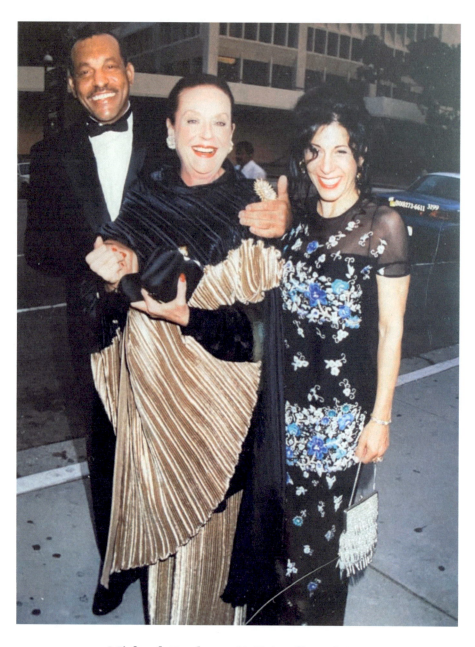

Michael, Barbara (A Friend) and Ava

CHAPTER NINE
SECOND ACT

The Second Act

The second act

Wants to explore what you've learned

You were on your path

When you suddenly turned —

Left and down,

Or "The Road Not Taken,"

But where you ended up

Left you lonely and shaken.

Life can break you down

But only to set you straight

If you let it — back to the path

You were always meant to take.

K.B. Hill

CHAPTER TEN

TOM MONE - THE MAN FROM EXETER

I parked under a bridge in downtown Los Angeles. It had been a long time since I was last in this area. Getting out of the car, I made a mental note of a few places to take a look at after this interview. I walked past an empty lot littered with trash and collapsed homeless tents. The building where I was to meet Tom Mone towered monolithically next to the lot. It was gated, with gardens planted along walkways, so I had to walk up and around the block to find the front entrance. Tom Mone is the CEO of One Legacy, the largest organ procurement agency in California.

Tom's second floor view was of the windows of other, taller buildings across the way, mostly empty streets in the waning, late autumn afternoon light. Because of Covid, Tom was appropriately masked up for our meeting, and I realized immediately that my interviewing skills were very much dependent on seeing people's faces. I could see his friendly blue eyes, almost twinkling, actually, as he greeted me. His hair was more white than grey and spoke to at least a part of his story. But I missed seeing his facial expressions. As I tried to write, it was becoming increasingly frustrating, as my glasses fogged up because of my own face covering. "How about this," he said, sensing my frustration, "I will move way back here, so we are really far apart, and we can take off our masks." He backed his chair up as far as he could. I tore the mask from my face and he removed his. A giant white mustache and a tiny soul patch surrounded a large, friendly smile. I love that he has a soul patch, because he saves souls. There was an instant warmth emanating from him that had been hiding behind that mask, and I felt almost transported back in time . . . not to just before Covid, but back to somewhere in another century. He has a gentlemanly quality that seems mostly lost on people today. There was an openness and kindness that put me instantly at ease. And, even though he had moved to California from Exeter, New Hampshire when he was only 12 or 13 years old, I could still feel the New England vibe. There is a European heritage in New England, unlike many other areas of the United States. Not quite at the Atlantic shoreline, Exeter does have many rivers and streams running through it. It is the birthplace of many dreamers and doers. David Chester French, the sculptor of the statue of Abraham Lincoln which graces and inspires the Lincoln Memorial in Washington, D.C. William Perry Fogg, an American author and adventurer, whose *Round the World: Letters from Japan, China, India and Egypt* (1872), was the inspiration for the character of Phileas Fogg in the Jules Verne novel *Around the World in 80 Days*, were both from Exeter, New Hampshire. And there it was. When Tom told me he had majored in Asian studies, I instantly saw it. Phileas Fogg — in the flesh!

He has travelled and continues to travel throughout Asia, and works with the Chinese government on the development of their donation program. The Chinese government, in an effort to create a more humanitarian program, stopped the use of organs from executed prisoners in 2015. "Organ donation must be completely altruistic, " he says. Tom, ever drawn to the history of Asia, sees China as the Middle Kingdom. That is to say, China keeps itself centrally controlled, and is becoming a mecca for art, literature, economic growth, understanding and prosperity, as was Egypt in its Classical Age. They want to rebuild the Silk Road. Not in a dark, cryptocurrency way, but with respect to world trade. "Less than one percent of us can be a viable organ donor, so it is — it must be — an act of humanity to make the decision to be a donor," he tells me. It is a difficult task, surely, to make the entire world understand and get on board with his thinking. "There are real world complications, and I have to help people move from wishful thinking to reality." Tom understands that for some communities that have a lower rate of donors, getting the countries of their origins to commit to this worldly sense of altruism is the key to getting that entire community to step up. "So, in Southern California, for example," he tells me, "where the Asian community has the lowest number of organ donors, getting Asian governments to conform to the North American standard of organ donation is critical." The Asian American community, like so many communities, follows the traditions and beliefs of its homeland. "Getting them to change is like a grassroots movement, backed by a global one." And for this man from Exeter, who majored in Chinese history at UCSB, Tom is uniquely suited to this particular aspect of his job.

Before we continue on the journey of Tom Mone's fascinating life, I ask how it all works. There are fifty-eight organ procurement operations in the United States, and, although, through the writing of this book, I have come to understand some aspects of organ donation, what is the actual order of things? I also bring up the subject of people being paid for, or worse killed, for their organs. It seems like a bit of a conspiracy theory, but it also seems to be a legitimate question. "In the United States," he tells me, "you can't just kill someone on the street and sell their organs to the nearest hospital. Not only would the hospital not accept it for ethical reasons, but the organ or organs also would not likely be viable. Less than 1% of us can be viable organ donors. Once someone is accepted as a donor, an entirely different medical process begins. It is a process to make the organs the best they can be for transplantation." If someone suffers a brain death, One Legacy gets a call. After a donor has been found, the hospital takes three or four days to try to improve organ function before the transplant actually takes place. "We get 70,000 calls per year, and only 1/10 of those are possible donors. Someone is sent out to assess, and if there is no active cancer, with the exception of some brain cancers, we can proceed. If there is active cancer, they cannot be a viable donor. If the donor patient is not registered, we go to the family." I think about my high school friend, Jon Stewart. We called him Poodle. He was absolutely the best of us, and as if 2020 wasn't difficult enough, we lost Poodle to cancer. But after he passed, the hospital approached his family to ask if he would be a cornea donor. Without hesitation, Poodle's family agreed. So for the two people, each of whom received one of his eyes, 2020 was an amazing year. Only Poodle could make 2020 great! "So what about corneas and donors who have cancer?" I ask him. "Corneas are always good," Tom says, smiling.

Personal stories make the biggest impact. There is a massive parade every year in Southern California called the Rose Parade. It has been going on for 130 years, as of 2020. One Legacy has a float in the Rose Bowl Parade. Tom's voice wavers a bit, as he talks about the floats. He is moved by the stories that are depicted on the float. I suppose I am one of those people who think floats are pretty and the work that goes into them is incredible, but as I learned, the stories behind the floats are the real gems. According to the One Legacy website, "Each year, Donate Life's lovingly crafted float features three categories of participants: Riders (all recipients of organs, tissues or corneas), Walkers (all living organ donors), and Floragraph Families (whose loved ones are depicted in dozens of memorial "floragraph" portraits of deceased organ and tissue donors) integrated into the float design. The float also features thousands of dedicated roses carrying messages of love, hope and remembrance." That float represents Life — in every imaginable stage. This year, when my husband puts on the Rose Parade, I will be watching it with a different set of eyes.

Originally, recipients were not allowed to meet donors. There is too much emotion. But when recipients began writing letters to donors, they found a human connection. Tom told me that when BBC reporter Reg Green's seven-year-old son, Nicholas, was killed in a botched robbery in Italy, he shared his son's story of being a donor. Donation rates went from 6.2 million to 20 million people. In an interview in 2017, Green said, "My son died in 1994, but his heart only stopped beating this year." While Tom does not necessarily believe in transference, it is that belief that sometimes brings a family to allow their loved one's organs to save the lives of others. And while he sees things from the point of view of an administrator, he believes that the whole world has the capability to come together to do this one thing — as a collective act of humanity. Each and every person can be a donor. When I ask him about God, as I do everyone I interview, he sits back and gives me that giant smile again. "We have no clue about God, so I'm not ruling Him out."

I ask him about Ava. "She's a real dynamo! She looks beyond herself. She has an entertainer's sense of self and she puts herself out there. She channels her energy to help other people." He knows that Ava's Heart needs to be a national program. When Dr. Mario Deng introduced them at a UCLA symposium, it was kismet. Ava had been looking to get more involved in helping transplant patients and had spoken to Jenna Rush to find out where the need was greatest. She had settled on post transplant housing. Upon meeting Tom, she found a kindred spirit in energy and drive to go out into the world and do something good that made a difference in peoples' lives. Of Tom, Ava told me, "He has this saying about his work and the world within it: 'This club is not one that anyone wants to join willingly, but once they do, they meet the most amazing people along the way.' And for me," she tells me, "It is an honor to call him my friend."

While Tom Mone understands the science of organ donation, he is also moved by the personal connection, life, and possibilities. *This* Phileas Fogg has done so much more than travelled around the world in eighty days. He is the man from Exeter who sees hope in every opportunity and sees opportunity in every corner of the world, to save a life, one soul at a time.

Tom Mone, the Man from Exeter

CEO of One Legacy

Believer in Humanity

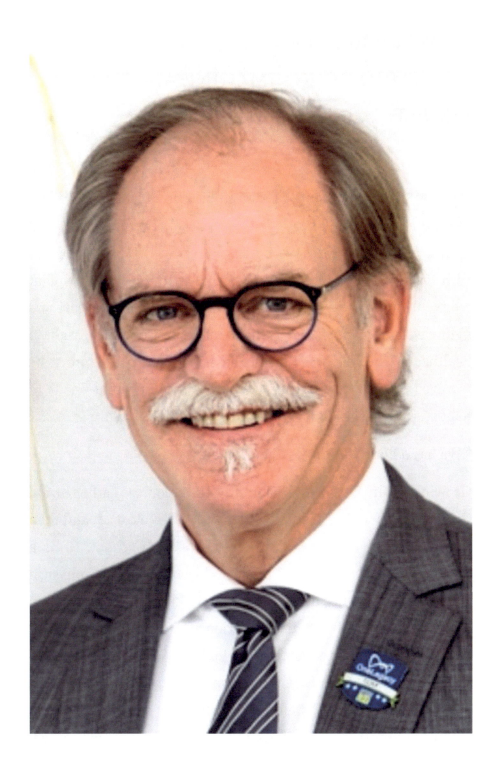

CHAPTER ELEVEN
DR. MARIO DENG - IMAGINE ALL THE PEOPLE . . . BEAUTIFUL DREAMER

Ava met Dr. Deng when UCLA hired him in 2011. Though it was clear that there had been some politics between Cedars and UCLA, like Ava, politics were not his concern. He watched her with the patients while he was working with a heart transplant recipient. After speaking with her, he knew that Ava's Heart was in line with his own vision of what healthcare was. "Basic right in healthcare," he told me, "means all healthcare people must be involved in the process to make sure everything that needs to happen for the patient is addressed."

"Ava has a beautiful professional vision."

Growing up in Berlin and Hamburg to a Chinese father and a German mother, Mario studied Latin at 10, Greek at 14, and then traveled to the United States in 1972 for high school. He is a beautiful human being. Not just because of his physical appearance but because of his vast knowledge and deep understanding of the human experience. I have personally met quite a few similarly educated people. In my experience, they go one of two ways. There are those who are incredibly book smart. They are educated and well-spoken and they see themselves as better than most people and hold themselves in very high regard.

And then there is the other kind of person who takes all of their knowledge and combines it with a spiritual understanding of humanity that transcends most societal restrictions. The latter is Dr. Mario Deng. He incorporates every aspect of his being into everything he does. For example, he does not, as a doctor, belittle the choice of someone to be an athlete. He had wanted to be a decathlete, and he took great knowledge from his years as an athlete himself. "I wasn't good enough to be a decathlete," he tells me. "So I went with my backup plan to be a doctor." And yet, he still draws on his experience as an athlete to help him understand and explain the limitless belief in the ability of the human body to overcome physical limitations to achieve excellence. He still sees himself from that other time in his life. "I believe essential spirituality governs life. I do not take myself out of the equation when I speak to my patients."

Mario sees being a person as sharing the space. He holds his patients' hands and connects with them when he talks about their health or that of a family member. "I need to be able to talk *with* my patients and cry with them." He tells me of an instance when he was sitting with a woman and her children. He had to tell them that her husband, their father, was going to die. "When a patient dies, it is a very personal experience. Sitting in a room with his wife and children, I take her hand and look into her eyes. We do not speak for twenty seconds. I do not have the right words yet. It is in this silence that I communicate the impending death. We do not need the English language at that moment. I must resonate with my own mortality. I am not in denial. Dying is part of living."

And so, in this utter silence, both doctor and patient's wife understood all of that. Mario sees, feels and lives the connection with other people — as he did with Ava — and as he does with patients and with other people in his life. His connection to his own wife, Federica, embodies this. He speaks about her like she is the other half of him. Federica is a professor of research who Mario met one day on a beach in Sandy Hook, New Jersey. She offered him a shaved carrot, and they spoke for three hours. She was in science education. "It was a wonderful, educated conversation." His eyes sparkle when he talks about her. Almost twenty years after that day on the beach, you can feel his adoration for her, blazing across the internet and into my dining room. As she enters the conversation, I see an extraordinarily beautiful woman with thick, dark, wavy hair that frames a face from a famous painting. I can't put my finger on it, perhaps because she is talking. Like Mario, she is so intelligent that I need to focus on her words. "Did Mario tell you he thought Ava was a spy?" She laughs. "Tell her the story!" And she nudges him. "I did. I thought she was a spy," he says. He is a little shy about it. "I said that nothing about the whole Cedars - UCLA thing was my concern, but maybe I was a little paranoid. I had heard Ava came from Cedars, and she was talking to everyone! The patients, the doctors. And everyone loved her. I thought maybe she was there to steal more people away and take them to Cedars." Federica laughs and comes front and center again. They are like two sides of a heart. One definitely functions better when they are both there. I find myself wishing I was actually sitting in the room with them, opening a bottle of wine and getting a little drunk. I would have a better excuse as to why I have some trouble following the conversation about molecular biology and immunology. "Do you know why I love Ava so much?" Federica jumps in again. "Because when we met, I could see she was disappointed that Mario was married. I love that we have the same taste in men!" And then, just like that, she jumps back into science and research. In an article published on Federica Raia in 2014 by Joanie Harmon, Federica talks about the book that she wrote with Mario, "Relational Medicine". She explains it like this: "Relational Medicine, i.e., the integration of body, science technology and personhood into one singular framework of practice and that this integration can mean the difference between life and death." It's a common theme that runs throughout the many interviews I have conducted for this book. Community. It immediately reminds me of Anurag, another incredible intellect, who said, "It takes a village to raise a person and it takes a community to heal one." There is the village, the community, of doctors and researchers, of family and friends, of the lives and experiences and of death as being part of that life. It is a beautiful, hopeful way to approach medicine, where they look at combining all of the marvels of modern medicine with the life and feelings of the patients who experience it. Mario specializes in Advanced Heart Failure, an ever-changing, always-evolving branch of cardiology. Understanding that the patient goes through massive life changes and has to accept mechanical devices or a transplanted heart as a new part of oneself can be traumatic, difficult, life-changing, life-affirming, life-altering . . . the point being that it depends on that individual. There is a level of support that has to happen for the patient's life to feel whole and successful again. Ava's Heart is a huge part of that community. I am again reminded of Anurag's interview, when he said that people would ask him how his surgery went, and he would think, *"the surgery?? You mean my heart transplant?* They took my heart out of my body and put someone else's heart inside of me! *I have someone else's heart sewn into my body!* It wasn't just surgery!"

These are not just surgeries. They are a life-changing event.

Mario is well-traveled, first working in Europe, then at Stanford, where he was excited to take a position, being that the first heart transplant had occurred there. Then he went back to Berlin, and then took a job at Columbia. He worked in post-operative research there, developing the Allomap test through molecular immunology to help rule out heart transplant rejection, bypassing the usual, painful method of the heart biopsy. It's a fascinating idea, that they could identify the absence of rejection by a blood draw of the recipient's white blood cells, then subject these cells to gene-expression profiling with DNA microarray technology. In other words, the white cells look for danger and attack the new cells, the transplant. There is an *imprint* of that attack on the 37,000 genes that are in the white blood cells, and the peripheral blood of white cells shows that imprint in a blood draw. Having three kids who grew up watching the *Twilight* movies, when Mario used the term "imprint", I, of course, thought about the werewolves "imprinting" on whomever they were to care for and love throughout their lives. Not the same, but actually, exactly the same, just for different reasons. It is an involuntary phenomenon in which the werewolves find their true soulmate in the movie. It is clear how Mario met Federica that day on the beach in 2002, and it is the mark made on the genes in the white cells to mark danger, therefore projecting that rejection is possible. Genius.

Understanding the role that the immune system plays in our overall health is the most significant stride in medicine and wellness. Outside influences, such as illness, stress, jobs, friends and family, all play into our health. They are instrumental in building a greater understanding of how much control we have over our own well-being. Having a community of support throughout our lives and even as we die creates a completely different experience than just going it all alone.

My conversation with Mario shifts to death. "When patients code, (when they die) there are the most beautiful descriptions . . . light that involves transitions . . ." They talk about them when they are brought back to life. He has experienced this many times with patients, being that he works with many patients with Advanced Heart Failure. He sees them before and after their surgeries and deals with them on a very personal level. "It seems that the leaving experience for these people is less traumatic. When they come back, they are wondering what's wrong with everyone." They are suddenly forced back into a body that isn't working when they are somewhere beautiful and peaceful and pain-free. I find comfort in his words. He is right that when we speak of death, I find myself thinking about my own demise, but I do not feel fearful about it. It almost feels like an exciting new adventure.

As I speak with this man I am so aware of Federica's part in his life. They understand life on a molecular level and how every part of our being, down to the single-cell that started us, is a part of a community. Without the rest of the cells, we cannot exist. And without a community once we are here, we cannot thrive. Using the parts of our brains that we may not be familiar with opens a vast world of knowledge and understanding, where we welcome the input of support from those who know what we are experiencing. Sometimes not using words, just looking into someone's eyes and holding their hand, communicates all that is needed. Mario has experienced this. His patients have experienced this. Federica watches and records and loves him so purely, that there is a comfort in knowing that kind of love exists. It's like he is standing naked in front of life, understanding that this is Life — from the first cell to the last breath.

Dr. Mario Deng

Soul Mate of Federica Raia

Imaginer of a Greater Community

Beautiful Dreamer

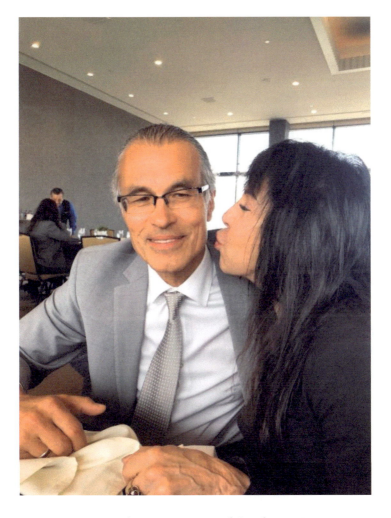

Dr. Mario Deng gets a kiss from Ava

CHAPTER TWELVE
THE FIGHTERS, THE SURVIVORS, AND THE SOULS THAT LIVE ON

The interviews with organ transplant recipients and organ donor families are not easy. Because they were conducted during the time of Covid, I could not hold any of them when they cried, or even touch them on the arm. I often sat with a person's story for a few days after the interview because my heart ached for them. To tell the story of someone's journey properly, I watched each person carefully. The shifting of eyes, trying not to cry, the wringing of hands when they felt helpless. Sometimes there was a far-off look, wishing that things had turned out differently.

We often look at organ transplants as "surgery" — but it's not just surgery. It is someone's chance at life again. When a recipient prays for a heart, lungs, liver or kidney — they do not wish for someone to die, though it might feel like that. And even the youngest recipients have to deal with the ramifications of what they have wished for. It is a complex wish, and sometimes the donor families don't want to ever meet the recipients of their loved one's life-saving organs. While this is hard for some of us, including me, to comprehend, we cannot judge it. One of the Donor Moms you will read about, knows every recipient of her son's organs. She has an especially close relationship with the recipient of her son's heart. When that young man started to have some rejection issues two years after he got the heart, he didn't want to tell the Mom. He feared she would feel like she was losing her own son all over again. The medication was adjusted, and he was okay again. These are exceptional people who remind us that the smallest things we take for granted, like walking up the street without labored breathing, a deep breath that fills every part of your body, would be a dream come true for them. A heart beating without pain, a body free of pain. Or even sight. Sometimes, the transplanted organ offers the chance to recapture lost youth or the chance to just feel "normal."

Some of these stories are about people with genetic disorders they were born with. Some, like Ava, are people who have medical problems thrust upon them. I don't know which is more profound a journey . . . to have been strong and lost it., and then fight like hell to get it back, or to feel strong or "normal" for the first time in one's life. These are the stories of how simple lives transcend the norms and become extraordinary stories. And more importantly, every single story offers hope.

After all, hope is the key . . .

To success . . .

To achieving dreams . . .

To living life.

To the survivors, the donors, and to everyone who has loved and lost among them, these are your stories. Your strength is astounding, your resolve is inspirational, and the hope with which you live every single day emboldens us to grasp firmly onto our own lives and make a difference.

CHAPTER THIRTEEN
JOE LAFFERTY - NOT DONE YET . . .

Ava first met Joe at the Donate Life Hollywood gala. He is a double transplant recipient, a kidney and a pancreas. He has such tremendous energy that, even in our video conversation, I can feel him flying a hundred miles an hour through my computer screen. Like I am about to hear a hilarious comedian do a set on stage. The very first time we spoke, he said something that struck me. "I'm not responsible for Justin's soul, but I am responsible for the time he's given me." Justin was his donor. Joe wrote a book called *Justin Time*. There is a picture of Justin that looks like anyone's son in a high school yearbook. From beneath a mop of chestnut brown hair, a handsome kid with a big smile, looks back at the page. He has broad shoulders and looks strong and athletic. He was 16 when he was killed in an accident. Staring at his photograph, it dawns on me how difficult this journey is going to be — talking to people like Joe because for every person who has received this life-saving gift, another has given that gift. I look at Justin again. Anyone's son . . . mine . . . yours . . . anyone's. And maybe that's the whole point of Ava's journey and Joe's journey, and everyone else I was going to meet. The selfless gift of life. The whole point is to say "yes", because there but for the Grace of God go any of us.

Joe smiled broadly as he spoke. His gratitude for his own life is palpable in every word. At one point as if it's not part of the conversation, he throws in, "...and then after I lost my eye...."

Stop.

"Joe," I say, "you lost your eye?"

"Yeah! Didn't I mention that?"

Nope.

Joe has a kid-like way of talking and looking at the world. His one eye dances about while he's talking. The conversation continues about his life and his transplant journey until another interjection: "after I survived cancer . . ."

What? I have to back up the conversation. "What did you say about cancer?"

"Oh yeah", he says. "When I was 8 years old, I had Non-Hodgkin's Lymphoma."

Oh yeah?? Like a side note to an already incredible story of survival. Joe had cancer when he was a little boy. He went through chemotherapy and radiation for a year and a half. He finally finished all of his treatments when he was ten years old. He had developed pancreatitis during the cancer treatments. He heard his father crying outside of his hospital room one night. He had been in so much pain, that he knew in his heart, that his father was crying because he knew his young son was going to die. Joe was nine at the time, and understood that. He made peace with it almost immediately, even as a small boy. His focus was more on his father's sadness than on his own mortality. But when Joe didn't die. His father came into his room, filled with resolve. "Okay! Here's what we're going to do next . . ."

Then, when he was thirteen, he found out he was an insulin-dependent diabetic.

I found myself taking a pause thinking about this young kid, being robbed of such a big chunk of his childhood to fight cancer, then getting sick from the treatment meant to get rid of cancer, then getting better. Beating cancer, only to find out he was diabetic.

He became "that kid who had cancer", instead of just being Joe. In the early eighties, compassion was not something that was taught in schools. But sometimes, there is an extraordinary kid, who understands that the fight he already fought will be so much harder than anything else he will ever have to do. No uneducated or intolerant comment could stop him from doing the things he loved. And he knows that the strength he'd garnered from experience was what would define him.

But God wasn't done with Joe yet.

When he was 29 years old, he was helping his friend's father restore a home in Texas. While cutting back some bushes, he got cut along the left side of his head above his ear. Over the next week, an infection set in, and he woke up one morning with an itchy eye. As the hours progressed that day, it began to throb. A friend took him to an optometrist, who immediately rushed him to an ophthalmologist, who in turn, rushed him into surgery at the local hospital. The doctors injected antibiotics, but a staph infection had set solidly in. Joe was told that his vision wouldn't likely return, and upon seeing his eye, he said, "it looked like someone had stirred my eyeball."

The doctors told him that if he didn't let them remove the eye, the staph infection would likely reach his brain and kill him. He put an open bible over his face and prayed for guidance. His eye was removed the next morning, and as Joe says it, ". . . and that's when I started life as a one-eyed person!"

It occurs to me here that Joe and Ava have more in common than their transplant stories. Ava too, is a single mastectomy cancer survivor, and she's had two hip replacements as well. I smile, and think to myself, that, I guess, after Ava's mastectomy, that's when she started life as one boobed person. Joe tells me that he would do just about anything to have two good eyes, not have a scarred-up body, and not have had to deal with cancer when he was a boy. Their scars are roadmaps to the warriors they have been.

Well, Joe's story is still longer.

At 31 years old, his organs began failing, and he had a pulmonary embolism. His kidneys stalled in January 2007, but re-started. In September of that same year, they failed again. By November, he was being examined to be put on a list for organs when they found out he had a heart problem. Two leaky valves had to be replaced, so that he could be put on the list for a kidney. After scores of medical issues, Joe finally got his heart surgery on July 25, 2008. That was a Friday. He didn't wake up until the following Thursday. Joe had flatlined after the surgery and was gone for seven minutes. I thought about Ava when she died. I wondered if Joe had a similar experience: smelling her daughter's dirty hair, getting her shark heart, and finally, promising God she would spend the rest of her life giving back if He would let her live. Joe said, "It's like the Footsteps poem: 'During your times of trial and suffering when you see only one set of footprints, it was then that I carried you.'"

Joe got the call for his organs in February, 2010. He was 37 years old. He was a soldier, fighting all the way, never losing faith that he would recover. He told me that he felt he spent much of his life lacking empathy, but I see him very differently. He lived those first 37 years intent on staying alive, never stepping away from the path that was laid out for him, and trusting that God had a plan beyond the next surgery. He finds strength in his family and in his religion — and it's absolute and unwavering.

Six months after Joe got his double organ transplant, he met Jennifer. Or, actually re-met. He had known her before through family. She is the love of his life. And when he wonders for even a brief moment why he had to wait so long for such pure love, he quotes the lyrics from a song by Fink:

And the things that keep us apart

Keep me alive

And the things that keep me alive

Keep me alone

Joe never doubted and God delivered with both hands.

Joseph Patrick Lafferty

Double Transplant Recipient

Lives *very* happily with the Love of his Life, the beautiful, green-eyed

Jennifer

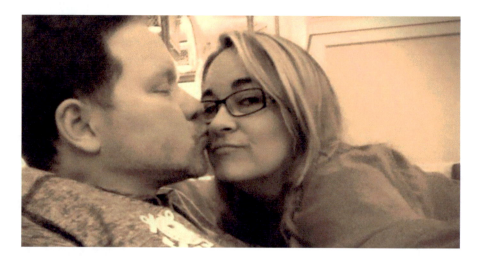

Joe Lafferty and the Beautiful Green-Eyed Jennifer

ADDENDUM
JOE, ON A MONDAY

It is a Monday morning in May of 2022. May 2nd. This book is actually at a publisher, where the page layouts are happening, and we are so excited to present everyone who participated with their own copy. Joe Lafferty is the head of Ava's board for Ava's Heart. He calls her daily, opening the call with, "Hey Boss!"

Ava laughs when she talks to him. He is so positive and it comes from him with such effortless ease – for someone who has been through everything he has had to endure. "Every single day," she tells me, "without fail – Joe sends me an inspirational quote to start my day. He sends one to me and he sends one to another friend and then he posts it on his Instagram. But he didn't send one today . . ."

At this very moment in our conversation, I am driving along the water between Santa Barbara and Ventura in California. It is the start of my long drive into work. There is so much construction on the road, and the wild waters of the Pacific Ocean are a gorgeous swirl of greys and blues. There are white caps as far as the eye can see – and I hit that autopilot feeling – where there are just your senses, following what you do every day – taking over for you. The ocean seems so vast – so neverending. And as I have so many times before, I imagine myself running to the edge of a cliff over the ocean and flying off in a beautiful swan dive. When

I hit the water, I become a mermaid and I swim away into eternity.

Eternity.

I never realized that when I wrote Joe's chapter, and he said to me, "God wasn't done with me yet", that God would need such a remarkable man closer to him – and that that time would come sooner than later.

Ava had sent Joe a text, asking for her inspirational quote for the day, and she got a response from Joe's sister to please call his mother. Her heart sank.

My heart sank.

"Joe passed away last night." Ava was so sad. She had such a wonderful friendship with him and he helped so much getting Ava's Heart into a better space. She didn't feel so alone, because he was giving her help and structure and support. Taking the calls she does everyday leaves a deep impression on her – the families who need a place to stay and the donor families, who are calling to get help to bury a son or daughter or husband or wife. It's a lot – and Joe knew that and he tried to take some of that pain from her.

I reached Ventura, and continued on, somehow arriving at my first appointment in West Hollywood. I don't remember the drive – over the big hill and down into the West Valley on the 101 freeway – through the canyon, lined with the hot pink bouganvillea and the low, wispy branches of the pepper trees – because I was busy imagining my eternal swim in the ocean.

Joe is out there, helping God make the ocean beautiful, breaking through the low hanging grey clouds with brilliant rays of sunshine. The sight is so spectacular, I want to pull over and take a picture. I know it's Joe. He can see out of both of his eyes again and God will tell him all about why he had cancer when he was a little boy. God will explain everything to him now.

The thing about grey days, is that they make all of the greens in the world look deeper and richer – like how the color green was always meant to be. Green is Life. And in the exquisite green eyes of Jennifer, the love of Joe's life . . . is reflected all of the depth – the richness – the endless life and energy – that was him.

Joseph Patrick Lafferty. You will be so very . . . eternally . . . missed.

CHAPTER FOURTEEN
CRAIG ERQUHART - INTO THE BLUE

Craig, or Seejai, was born in Detroit, Michigan. It strikes me the number of athletes I have met who are from Detroit. It's like every other person I meet who is exceptional at their sport is from Detroit. And in Seejai, I again encounter that zest for life. That if his first dream couldn't happen, he was just going to go after the next thing, seemingly unfazed. He has a smooth, calming voice when he speaks, even when it is about his medical history. He reminds me of the World War II vets who have a veritable laundry list of accomplishments post-war. He started a foundation and mentors kids, has a clothing line and is a musician. Ava met Seejai at a Christmas party for transplant patients at UCLA. A doctor introduced them by saying, "Ava, I want you to meet Seejai. He actually had the same thing you did." She felt an instant connection.

Seejai grew up with both parents, his brother, and his sister — spanning the eighties and nineties, as a six-foot, six-inch tall basketball player who was NBA bound. But his "episodes" sidelined him with enough consistency, it was suggested that he wear a heart monitor.

"It's a chest pain — but from the inside — like someone pounds and pounds on your chest from the inside, trying to get out. It

feels like it's so badly bruised on the inside, I would need to lie very still and wait for it to stop — sometimes for hours."

But Seejai didn't want anything to do with a heart monitor. He ignored his "episodes", because they represented an athlete having to stop, and that just wasn't him.

His first episode happened in the seventh grade, and they continued until he sought treatment almost twenty years later. He was a giant of a man, stuck in a body that wasn't obeying his commands. Everything about him — his spirit and his height and his drive and understanding of the sport — *all* said: "Go!" But the bruised, pounded-upon chest said, "Stop!" The episodes would continue throughout high school and would plague him at every college tryout. He was told he had Arrhythmia and that he had Endocarditis. Arrhythmia can manifest as a heart beating too fast or too slow. It can be described as "fluttering". It can go away on its own or can be a symptom of a more serious condition. Endocarditis is an infection of the endocardium, which is the inner lining of the chambers and valves of the heart. It can be caused by bacteria getting into the heart, and can be fatal if not treated by antibiotics. Neither of these was his problem. To him, the fact that he couldn't pass the physical exams was the *only* problem. Seejai continued to push it all aside, insisting on achieving the athletic excellence he knew was his birthright. Eventually, he was recruited by Tennessee, played for Ohio Junior College, then transferred to Eastern Michigan. His junior year at college was "hazy". He had to do a treadmill test, which marked his heart rate at 195, so once again, he couldn't pass his physicals. He had reached a level of success, pushing as hard as he could. But the sleeping giant in his chest would bring him to the floor, where he would lie, in a seemingly swirling repetition of pain, quietly calming his body. He couldn't run far enough from it, or jump out of it.

Once he accepted that a basketball career was out of reach, Seejai moved to Los Angeles and started his music career. He sings in style he describes as "alternative soul: R & B meets Phil Collins". Listening to his voice, it belongs to a young man, who is filled with hope for himself and for the world. In the video of one song, he sings, amidst images of his transplant surgery and his first steps post-surgery, "*All I wanna do is move on, and All I keep telling myself is be strong . . .*" It is the story of inspiration, strength and resolve. This is a man who never backed down, and whose body held out as long as it could.

Seejai has died twice. In the span of *twenty years* of a misdiagnosed heart condition, living with a pain that came to be normal for him, his heart actually died. And at that moment, he floated above himself on the table, with medical staff working on him - talking to himself. He watched from above as the people who were working to bring him back all seemed to morph together into the most beautiful blue hue he had ever seen. He was aware of each person, but they were energy, not human forms. And he knew he had to go back. As the paddles shocked his heart again and again, he slipped back into his bruised body. The beautiful blue faded away, and he awoke.

He couldn't completely describe the blue, except to say that it represents the sky, the sea, and calmness, as the color blue goes. A blue aura is said to reflect humanity's calmest tendencies. Tranquility and relaxation. People who have that aura are compassionate and intuitive and are deeply in tune with their voices. It is reflected in the thyroid and throat area of the body and is said to reflect honesty, self-expression, good speech and communication. All of those qualities are Craig Erquhart. He speaks calmly, always with a slight smile. His eyes dance a little when he talks about the beautiful blue and about his wife, Keesha and his brother, Brandon. They pulled him through his four-month stay at Torrance Memorial Hospital and then his seven-month stay at UCLA. They encouraged him through four-and-a-half months of having a life-saving device called a "bi-vat" inserted into his body. "*That*", he said, "is a whole different kind of pain I can't even describe, except to say that I wouldn't wish it on my worst enemy."

Seejai's donor was a young man whose story is not his, or mine, to tell. But I will say this: he was also an athlete with an imposing physique, just like Seejai's. He was 33 years old when he died and when he gave Seejai back a life he hadn't had for twenty years. But in his donor's life, there was one more journey that Seejai became a part of.

A heart is a funny thing. If you look it up in a medical book, you will learn about the muscle that is your heart, and its chambers and valves. You will learn about its function in the human body. But what you *won't* see, is how the heart has a life that is attached to your emotions. When someone breaks your heart, there is a physical pain in your chest. When you achieve something amazing, your heart will flutter with excitement. It is as alive with your life, your loves and your achievements as much as your brain is, and as much as the words you can scream when you win a race or get an award or fall in love for the very first time. We've all been there — maybe only once — maybe several times — but every human being on the planet knows their heart travels with them throughout their life, be it short or long, be it one of need or pain, or one of riches and plenty.

After Seejai's heart transplant, he walked through his life, slowly — deliberately — but with the constant feeling that he was being watched. He concentrated on the presence, and eventually heard a child's voice: *"Where are you?"* Never one to turn down someone in need, Seejai contacted his donor family and asked about a child who would be calling for his donor. He knew that the beating heart in his body was calling to someone and that someone — a child — heard his voice. The family told him that his donor's very best friend was his eight-year-old nephew, who continually looked for him after his passing. With that knowledge, Seejai knew his heart could rest. His donor's nephew knew that his uncle was in good hands. He knew that he was allowed to see and hear the child because that little boy needed closure.

Seejai has a strong sense of faith, and together with his wife Keesha and his brother Brandon, his belief in a higher purpose pulled him through a life of unbelievable pain. Being an athlete gave him the drive to never give up.

Never give up.

Breathe — And Just Keep Walking

Into the Blue.

Craig "Seejai" Erquhart

Heart Transplant Recipient

Lives happily with his wife, Keesha in Los Angeles

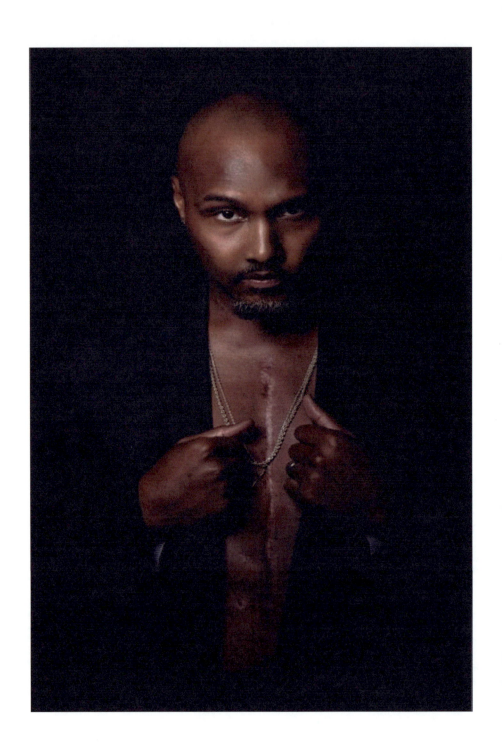

CHAPTER FIFTEEN
CAMERON BOLTON & SARAH FISHER - OVER THE RAINBOW

Ava met Sarah Fisher when Sarah reached out to tell her she loved what she was doing with Ava's heart. They started a conversation and Sarah told Ava her story . . . Cameron's story.

As a mother, this is a particularly difficult chapter to write. In fact, I kept putting it off, because Sarah's voice over the phone broke my heart. When she spoke to me about Cameron, I could only picture my own son, who is a few years younger and of a similar spirit. Cameron loved to go ATV riding, like my son loves his motorcycle. Everyone he met, said Sarah, knew they had a friend for life in Cameron. My son still keeps in touch with friends from kindergarten, even though we have moved many times. Cameron was energetic, adventurous and fearless. He liked fast toys, like snowmobiles, motocross bikes and remote control cars. I kept remembering my little boy, from the age of two, in his Spiderman pajamas, transfixed by his Hot Wheels, making race car sounds as he parked, hundreds of them, under every piece of furniture we had. Sarah lived with fear somewhere in her mind that Cameron would be hurt doing one of the things he so loved. I have that same feeling and her words are foreboding for me. As my son works across the table from me, fixing a Go-Pro camera to his motorcycle helmet, telling me about his "life dream" of being a vlogger on his bike, my stomach trembles inside.

I finally got to speak with Sarah on a video chat. As the picture opens up, I see a beautiful, petite woman, with dark blonde or light brown hair —I never really know the difference — lean, defined shoulders, on which she carries the world, and deep, tired eyes that have not stopped crying for a little over two years. She excuses herself for not wearing make-up but says she knows it will only run because of her tears. My eyes see far beyond that. I do not see a woman who needs makeup. I see a mother who raised this young young man, who we would all be proud to have raised. He was a reflection of her, and she now carries his legacy with her everywhere. It is the strength she shows in her resolve to make sure he is never forgotten — it is in every tear that falls from her eyes — it is in what she wears and in how she speaks. He does live on, because she makes sure of it.

Cameron was an "all-boy" little guy, with a big smile and wide-set eyes that sparkled with a touch of mischief. Sarah told me that they would never come home from the grocery store or other errands without a new toy tractor or another piece of farm equipment so that Cameron could put together his own farm. It was *his* farm, and he didn't feel he needed to share his operation with either of his siblings. He designed an entire working farm, and played with it, mesmerized by the imaginary world he had created. He was bothered only by two things: the tags inside his shirts, and the seams on his socks. He would refuse to wear the socks, claiming that they were "broken", because he didn't like the feeling of the seams on his toes; Sarah would find the offending socks tossed in the corner of the closet at some later time. His Grandma came to live with the family and, at just two years old Cameron took it upon himself to be a perfect little gentleman to her, holding open doors and showing her love and kindness whenever he had the chance. They remained close until her death when he was a sophomore in high school. Cameron's heart was always in the right place, and it was big enough to share with everyone he met. It is said that children, being newly from heaven, know and understand love better than those of us who have been here longer, but Cameron never lost that purity.

Cameron began driving real farming equipment by the age of seven, and after high school, he worked at a local family farming business. Along the way he developed a love for snowmobiles and BMX bikes. Anything fast. He would make piles of dirt for four-wheeling around the yard with his friends. Sarah gets a distant look in her eye and smiles, slightly, as she describes Cameron's first car which wasn't a car at all. It was a giant truck, with giant tires, that she needed a ladder to climb into. Cameron straight-piped the muffler, to make sure everyone would know he was coming. I am listening to her speak, knowing that kid so well, not wanting to have to continue with her story. I know where it's going, and I feel as though I want to stop the story here — to keep him that funny, sassy, smart, kind young man. I don't want to get to the next part.

As I am writing this, I occasionally stop to sift through the photos that she sent me. Cameron's spirit jumps off the images at me, always smiling, holding his family, loving his niece, Ezra. Looking out from under a construction helmet, he leans against a wall, standing proudly in front of his "giant, straight-piped" white truck, holding a snowsuit-clad Ezra, as easily as if she had been his own child.

He smiles, he smiles, he smiles.

Sarah was watching the news in late June, 2018, when there was a report of a fatal car crash outside of Fargo, and she thought, "I have to pray for that family." Two hours later, she got a call from the hospital — the only trauma center in the area — where she works as a certified nursing assistant. I cannot imagine her ride to the place where she had seen so many others brought in for life-saving procedures. I know she took in the information she was given, but she prayed for a miracle. Cameron was declared brain dead, and yet, his heart beat on. That big heart that built a farm operation. That big heart that loved an aging grandmother and treated her with reverence. That big heart that enveloped his family and friends and loved a smitten niece — that big heart that wouldn't let go . . . .

Because it had more work to do . . .

Only one percent of hearts are viable as donor's hearts. With no heartbeat, a heart cannot be viable. But, while Cameron's heart did stop beating at the scene of the accident, paramedics worked tirelessly on him and were able to get a heartbeat back. It took them twenty minutes — but during that twenty minutes, his brain had been deprived of oxygen, and was unable to live. His hospital room was covered in crosses, and filled with the prayers of his family and friends. Sarah needed to live in a state of hope that Cameron would wake up, but it wasn't going to happen. She knew that, somewhere deep inside her own heart. She felt him leave and she knew how he would have wanted to give of himself. She told me that at the moment the family decided to donate Cameron's organs, a huge rainbow filled the sky above the hospital. Again, he enveloped her with his love and everything beautiful this life had to offer — all the colors in the rainbow. And on the day of the donation, something amazing happened. Ezra, Cameron's sweet little niece, who normally napped from one to three o'clock in the afternoon, awoke at 2:30 and announced to her nanny, "I know Uncle CeCe is okay now." As I said, children are closer to God, because they are fresh out of Heaven. It doesn't matter what you believe in. We are sometimes fooled into thinking they speak nonsense, but the words of a child are spoken with a deeper meaning that we can begin to understand.

Cameron Bolton visited his little Ezra while she napped, so she could tell everyone he was going to be okay. And he saved five lives the day he died. In the spirit of each of the people he saved, there's perhaps a little more "boy" spirit than there had been — perhaps one of them will look twice at farming machinery and have a deja vu of Cameron's long ago "farm operation", or when one of them is riding a bike, feeling the wind in their hair, they will pedal a little faster, getting a rush from the sound of the wind as they outrun it. And when each of them sees a rainbow, they will know that Cameron is just saying "Hi! I'm okay. Get out there and enjoy your day . . ."

Live. Love. Laugh.

Give life. Give love. Give laughter.

Donate.

Cameron Bolton

Donor

Died on July 2, 2018

. . . and lives on . . .

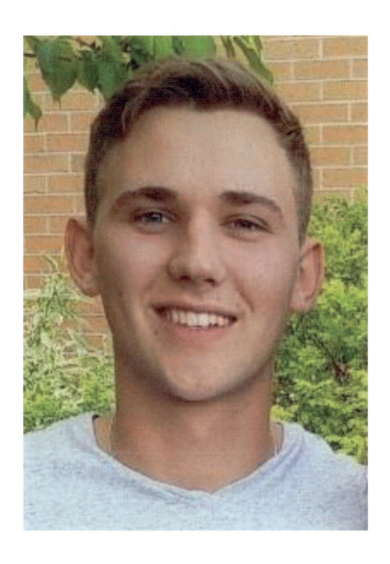

Cameron Bolton

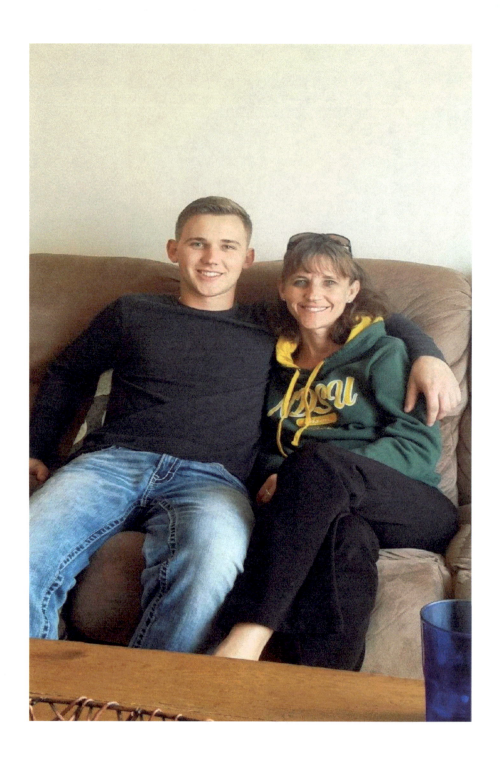

CHAPTER SIXTEEN
THE HIDING PLACE

The Hiding Place

A place where the skies last forever
And the wind blows high and free
My emotions run wild through the air and the trees
A place that waits for me . . .

There are no bars on the windows there
Upon a cliff over the sea
A castle from ages and ages long past
If you're looking, that's where I'll be

White-winged horses wait for the wind
To catch a gust — to fly!
I soar with them into Eternity
Time doesn't matter — Pass it by!

Here I know, this could be Infinity

Alive — through all the ages

The secret — the answer — lies locked in your heart

Not on any pages

Find Life

Within

Yourself . . .

K.B Hill

CHAPTER SEVENTEEN
FORGIVING FAMILY . . . OR NOT

Ava:

I write this tentatively. It has taken me some time to come around to my true feelings about my family and even some of my friends. There is so much pain wrapped up in my feelings about this. They say you can't choose your family, but you can choose your friends — and that I did — with a very open heart. I had friends from my dancing days and friends from working days and friends from the barn where Jade rode horses. I was like the mayor of Everytown, meeting new people and developing fast friendships and interesting acquaintances, and I was always comfortable with myself — no matter the situation. With my dancer fluidity I moved from circles of celebrities, to business people, friends of different religions, races and cultures, to the people who helped out at the barn and to the person standing in line for coffee at a cafe. I was just me — which is why it came as such a blow, when the betrayals of my family and friends began to reveal themselves. Like a child, I trusted the people I surrounded myself with and even more deeply, with family. As my illness robbed me of my home, security, and even my marriage, so did it rob me of that blind trust. People disappeared — people stopped calling and checking on me — I wonder if they even asked about me at all. Four months in the hospital, and not so much as a peep from my "best" friends. I was fighting for my life with every ounce of my being. Everything I had known outside of the walls of Cedars Sinai Hospital was crumbling and crashing to the ground. And people I had spent countless hours of my life with — laughing, sharing meals, gossiping at the barn, or chatting about anything and everything on the phone — were falling away. It wasn't even one by one. Sometimes it was a couple or a few at a time. While I fully understand that people need to move on with their own lives, this mass exodus of friends came as quite a blow.

The family dealt a crueler blow. At first, I thought I would keep my family business off the pages. These pages were sacred to me and to my work, but my journey brought me to a different place. Through my foundation, I have met so many incredible families. I found myself longing for the unconditional love that these families have for each other. I had heard, through my disappearing friends, that while I lay in the ICU at Cedars, with an L-vat, an R-vat, and a machine that breathed for me, with my dead heart and my crumbling life, my sister was telling anyone who would listen, that I never played by the rules. How I "always lived beyond my means". Did she believe that was a justification for my death?! Some friends seemed to accept that this perception of me, borne out of childhood jealousy, was a reason to abandon me. While I was held prisoner in a dark coma, people were excusing themselves from my life. And my sister felt vindicated for it.

What I realized — much later — was that she harbored deep-seated anger toward me for transgressions that I was completely unaware of. For leaving our family and pursuing a dream that she had long since abandoned. For loving and marrying my true love. For building a business and making my own money and acquiring things I wanted to have around me. Mona had carried hurt, anger and jealousy inside of her since she was a pre-teen. It festered and with every bad thing that happened to her, an illness grew with equal force. I admit that I enjoyed the wealth Michael and I had built up. But we built it through hard work, long hours, physical labor, relationships, never saying "no", being pushy sometimes, but being kind and respectful to everyone. Always. Did she not understand that?

I lived beyond nothing but my imagination and my wildest dreams. That bothered people.

I write about this because it, too, was a part of my recovery. Coming to terms with knowing that recovery was mine alone to deal with was tough, albeit necessary to get on with my life. Friends do pick sides in divorces and family does harbor resentment, perhaps more so in the face of impending death. I don't pretend to understand that, but I did come out of it knowing that I would not let other people feel that way.

Blue Skys grew so fast that we needed to buy a warehouse. My Uncle Saul invested a portion, but Michael and I invested the bulk of the purchase. It was our nest egg — that warehouse for our business. When the business was ready to sell, Saul would get his investment back — with interest — and Michael and I would have made a sizable profit from the sale. But life threw us a few curveballs. When I got sick, the company began to lose value, as did our home. But the warehouse — that was different. My uncle sold the building for a huge profit. If we had split the sale per our original deal, Michael and I would have sold the house, gone our separate ways, and had enough money to live on. But that's not what happened. My uncle kept all of the money, and doled it out to me as he felt I needed it. And Michael lost everything.

As of the writing of this book, my Uncle Saul passed away, well into his nineties, And my sister, my beautiful play doll who looked so much like me, that sometimes people would do a double-take — and yet was so unlike me — succumbed to brain cancer in 2019, at the age of 65. While compassion and kindness had long since seemed to have abandoned her, when I saw her before she passed away, I couldn't bring myself to show her anything but love and empathy for her pain. Throughout my journey with Ava's Heart, meeting such incredible families, I yearn for the love they have for one another. My eyes fill with tears when I think about who Mona was to me, and the trajectory of our lives from our home in Yonkers to our last moments together. Even in the end, with everything that happened, she will always be my baby doll. She left me without a word. No acknowledgment of who we once were. Although that is very painful for me, I know it must have been even worse for her. It was a lot to hold inside.

Until the day he died, Saul sat in his house, from his point of view, in a self-righteous state of mind, which brings me to another thing I learned in all of this.

Karma.

I no longer believe in karma, as I understood it in my other life. In the Buddhist definition, I suppose that what I do, have and am today could be the result of actions I took in past lives. But in the more Americanized/Christianized definition, it is that where I am now is a result of the life I lived up until this point. Babies who need heart transplants have done nothing to "deserve" the journey they will now have in their tiny lives. They do not "deserve" a life of medication and restrictions they will have to live with always. They have done nothing wrong. When I see the suffering of those tiny lives and those of their parents, I can no longer believe in karma. And as for Saul, while I must admit that I do not know his heart, I know that he loved his sister, my mother, with everything in him. Did he feel this way all along but behave himself while my mother was still alive? Or was he angry about losing her and was somehow taking it out on her children? He did not approve of me, but I really never found out why. Was it my marriage to Michael? Who knows the musings of an old man . . . to him, his idea of paying rent for me for a maximum of six months post-recovery was the appropriate time for "tough love" was so intensely out of touch, I had to shut myself off from the anger it made me feel. The thing was, at that point, I couldn't figure out up from down. I needed more than just a place to live. The anti-rejection meds made me shake and my hair was falling out — or maybe it was growing in — I couldn't tell. Food tasted different. Walking felt foreign. I felt like I was floating through a dream, and as I moved through it, I just wanted to find a way to wake up. I wanted to move and dance, and read and meditate. I had to go to rehab several times a week and often lacked the patience for the baby steps they kept wanting me to accept. (Give me a leap across the stage! Don't ask me if you can turn the treadmill up to 2.2 mph!!) I needed a job. I needed a purpose but I didn't know who I was or what I could do anymore. I used a walker and needed help with the simplest tasks. Where is the karma in learning to walk again? No one deserves this. As thankful as I was to be alive, holy shit was it hard!

But I can say that on the "other side" of all of that, I am able to make some small difference in people's lives. Perhaps, had Saul not robbed us of our livelihood, I would not have started this foundation . . . but there is no karma in any of that. There is, however, gratitude and there is the ability to cherish life with a greater appreciation of what I used to have. And I have always been grateful for my life, my strength and my family and friends. When I got out of the hospital, Clare came to stay with us. Beautiful Clare, who had her own life to deal with, but put everything on hold and came to help me reconnect to the world. Not many people are that pure of heart. In my view, there was

Mother Teresa, then Gandhi, then Clare — not necessarily in that order.

It was while I was in that apartment, that I got the news that my Daddy had passed away. I wasn't allowed to travel yet, being six months post-transplant, so I never got to see him again.

There's no kama in that.

Six months — six months — It was like a goddamn fly buzzing in your ear!

And the lease was up. It was time to move out.

Clare had to leave us. Even saints have lives they must return to. So there I was with my young child, trying to figure out where we could go to be safe and have a home. At first, we stayed with a friend and her daughters, but to my utter surprise, a thirty-year friendship crumbled in front of me. We lived on a ranch out in Fillmore, California. But, again at the whim of the homeowner, who was . . . well . . . we had to move on. I sometimes felt like everyone had abandoned me— not just me, but for Jade and me. Was it just too hard for them to see me in this state? It was not an easy or pretty recovery — but it was a recovery. I felt as though I was dragging my child with me through the worst part of my life — and she went willingly, with no complaints. She was as displaced as I was. And probably just as scared. I needed to take care of her, but before I could do that, I also needed to heal myself. I was having a hard time doing that with no job or money or place to call our own. I was in a fog. I had to find a way to dance again. That was number one. It was my connection to my own soul, which seemed to have gone on a vacation somewhere. And all the while, Jade watched, and we found her horses to ride. She grew taller and quieter. She continued to come home with that same dirty hair that brought me back to life. And then I remembered the promise I had made to God, as the doctors put the shark's heart into my chest, to spend the rest of my life giving back.

And there it was. Purpose.

I needed a home, where there was none . . . People needed a home during and after their transplants. People needed help with their medication. And donor families sometimes needed help cremating their loved ones.

It took months to set up my non-profit. It's mission: fill a need for others who were going to go through an experience like mine. Giving back was going to be a way for me to fill an empty spot. I realized that it wasn't my marriage . . . or my house . . . or the business . . . it was the deafening absence of my family. To this very day, that feeling can creep back inside me and try to penetrate my beautiful new heart. My parents were gone. A lifetime of camaraderie I'd had with Mona was gone. Her broken heart never got replaced. She lived with it. I think she may even have been envious that I got a new one.

To this very day as I write this story — deciding (slowly) what to share, or how much to say, the loss of my family still makes me cry. But I have learned that I do not have to cry only when I am alone in the shower. I am now surrounded by people who do not look at tears as a sign of weakness. The tears are shed when I watch families gather, support, and pray for their family member who is getting a transplant. They are shed because I miss my family and what I thought we were. In my family, money and jealousy won out over love, kindness and compassion. It might break my new heart a little, if I would let it, but I now choose to bask in the love these other families have for each other.

Karma.

CHAPTER EIGHTEEN
ANURAG SAKSENA - FROM INDIA WITH LOVE

I know for a fact that someone's heart can break more than once in a lifetime. This chapter is about how the power and workload of a man are matched by his unrivaled intelligence. The words he speaks and the way he thinks are a testament to the best that humanity has to offer. Anurag is one of the most fascinating and likely the smartest person I have ever met. He contacted Ava for help with housing, because, like so many other people in the transplant world, he was unaware that he would be required to have three months of post-transplant housing near the hospital. His situation was a little different than some of the other people who had stayed at Ava's House. He had the means to be able to secure housing, but there was a mold issue in the house he and his wife had rented, so he was introduced to Ava. He was in need of not only his second heart transplant, he also needed a kidney transplant. As soon as she finished speaking with him, Ava called me. "You have *got* to meet this man!"

 Something about Anurag resonated with me. I don't know if it was how intelligently he chose his words, or if it was his soulful brown eyes that looked like they brimmed with a well of stored up tears from a lifetime of adversity. I wanted to talk to him for hours and hours. His heart had broken more than once and his description of how it affected him made me feel like I was living it with him.

"I want you to understand something," he tells me. "My story is filled with adversity — with pain — but it is a story of triumph. Please know that. *It is a story of triumph.*"

Anurag, translated, means Love. He grew up in India in the 1960s in a family that was not wealthy. When I used to think of India, I imagined places like the Taj Mahal, Jaipur, the pink city, or Jodhpur, the blue city. I imagined the stunning and exotic places that I'd seen in pictures. I did not imagine that, within the view of the open windows of the colorful little villages built into stunning hillsides, there were people living in abject poverty. A friend of mine told me, upon her return from India, that I should not go there, because the children trying to sell me chewing gum on the street would break my heart. Their clothes were the colors seen in the most beautiful flowers in nature, but they concealed a pain shared by millions. And it is within such a dichotomy, that I understood the broken heart of this extraordinary man. After he finished school, Anurag left India to pursue a doctorate in Quantum Physics at the University of Manitoba in Winnipeg, Canada. He left behind his family and all of the customs and traditions that belonged to a life he was expected to live. There may not be a more unique place on earth than his home in Mathura, a sacred city in Northern India. But Anurag had an understanding of both the essence of quantum physics and its relationship to his own life, which drove him to leave India. He stowed that heritage deep inside, and crossed the world in pursuit of something else.

He met and married his wife, Manuela. She was from the Philippines, not part of his tradition or customs, now making the prospect of returning home an untenable choice. Without massive successes under his belt, he knew he would be looked at as a failure, so he stayed away. As much as he missed his family, he felt he could never return unless he did so with immense success.

The Winnipeg winters, when the temperature drops to forty below zero, are a kind of cold that is difficult to comprehend. "We were so poor," he tells me, "I could not afford to get myself or my family coats for winter." When he finally could put enough money together he bought coats for his wife and baby daughter. He, himself, wore a large sweatshirt, which he stuffed with newspaper to try to keep warm. I grew up in that cold. Those temperatures often lasted at least four months of the year. The sunset before four o'clock in the afternoon, giving way to frigid nights of deep, frozen snow, jagged icicles hanging from bare trees and air so cold that the hair in your nostrils would freeze over in less than a minute. It was incredibly beautiful to look at, but brutal to live in. Not unlike India, I suppose.

Anurag found work in the insurance business in Winnipeg, establishing the asset-liability program that all insurance companies now operate under. More work opportunities came to him after that, moving to Toronto, then Minnesota, New York and eventually settling in Washington D.C. They were doing very well, financially, but the stress of his work and spending fifty percent of his time travelling away from his growing family was a heavy burden. He was in the office, when, at 44 years old, he had a massive heart attack. His assistant found him. The paramedics arrived. As they worked tirelessly on him, he could hear their questions, but he couldn't respond. When they were at the hospital and the nurses ripped his shirt open, he finally spoke for the first time, telling them, "My wife is not going to be very happy that you ripped my shirt."

Anurag had two stents put in, but the scarring was so extreme on his heart, that the doctors told him they would not work well for very long. That was in February, 2006.

I asked Anurag what he attributed his heart attack too? "Sure," he said to me, "the stresses of my job were incredible. I was responsible for thousands of employees and billions of dollars worldwide. That comes with some stress. And stress accumulates in your body and it stays with you." There was a heartbreak with so many of the little things that happened while he served in his executive position at Freddie Mac. Sometimes it was the lack of respect, the knowing that there were people who would never take him seriously as an executive, their superior, or even as a man. He is quick to point out to me that heartbreak is not a medical term. I realize that, of course, but the heart is an organ that feels pain when you are sad. It's that tightness in your chest when you hear you have lost a close friend. It's the fluttering that happens when someone you love walks past you. It's not medical, but that doesn't mean it's not real.

I tried to imagine what it had been like for Anurag to leave his home in India. Knowing that his life was calling him away from the family he cared for so deeply. Was that his first heartbreak? His parents came from different backgrounds. His father was poor, while his mother was quite well off. She was fifteen years old and went from having a 24-hour butler to having nothing. Growing up, there were days when they didn't have enough to eat, but dinner was always a celebration of life and family. "I have tremendous regard for my parents," he tells me, "but once I broke tradition and left home, I could not use them as a resource."

Moving to the United States moved him even further from his culture. He was under a great deal of pressure at work. He was splitting his time almost equally between job and family. "The job stress," he says, "was second to the cultural shock. Don't take this wrong — I don't mean to be insulting," he told me, "but the people who worked for me for all of those years — the white people — they didn't like taking orders from a brown man. They just ignored me."

Heartbreak. To have worked so hard and to see the world through the eyes of quantum mechanics, just to be disregarded for the color of his skin. It gave injustice a whole new meaning.

When he had his first heart attack, he learned a lesson about his American friends. He learned that people didn't really want to know how he was feeling or what was going on. They didn't want to hear his perspective on his heartbreak. They wanted to drop off flowers while he was asleep or leave messages on the phone. They knew he wouldn't answer. No one was going to come to sit with him and just let him talk.

Anurag was on so many medications that he felt they were poisoning him. They made his heart go faster, just like his life, which, in turn, shortened the time a heart can live. His doctor told him, "You are going to need a new heart."

It's difficult to say whether or not Anurag did things for all the right reasons. A man who feels that he cannot return to his home in India, without incredible success, will seek that success — perhaps beyond reason. But this was a man whose name *meant Love*. And perhaps, had he simply spoken what was in his heart, exactly as he had felt it, his family would have taken him in without question. This is only my personal thought. My wish, perhaps. The norms and expectations that Anurag holds in his heart and soul differ greatly from those I can understand. And he looked to those cultural expectations to make sense of what he was going through. The customs he had turned his back on became the customs he craved. His mother passed away in 2012, while he was waiting for a transplant and his father died in 2014, while he was recovering from it. His eyes fill with tears when he talks about his parents. "Maybe they never forgave me for not being there, but I never told them about the transplant." Perhaps, much of what has caused Anurag such anguish in his life lies in moments of deciding *not* to speak. He tells me that every time he would write to his father about a big job he got, his father would tell him, "You sold yourself out." I cannot begin to imagine how to rectify that in my mind — or in my heart, for that matter. But I do think that as parents, we see a trap door through which our children will fall, and we try to stop them before that happens. Maybe that's what his father meant. Maybe he just wanted Anurag to stop and look at what was important. Had there been a conversation, I cannot help but hope that they would have understood each other. Manuela also sacrificed a lot — for her husband and for their children. If it had not been for her, he said, he would never have been able to finish his doctorate. "All of this was my journey. All of this stuff brought me to where I am now — and there is tremendous heartache in what I gave up — and tremendous love for what I gained."

To be on the receiving end of racism, when you have gone through everything Anurag had so far endured in his life — his poverty, his brilliance — his love of a woman who was not chosen for him through his culture. Writing a thesis that won so many accolades. But never being able to use that to any advantage. Starving. Freezing. Then finally working his way up to a position that he deserved, only to have employees disregard him for his brown skin . . .

I will say this. If you have never walked in the shoes of the person for whom you have such disdain, you cannot possibly understand them and should therefore not reveal to them even an ounce of your ignorance.

Kindness is free.

When he finally got his first heart transplant, on September 22, 2013, he wanted to reach out to his friends. He needed to tell people how he felt. When someone would ask him, "When is your surgery?" it almost felt like an insult. *His surgery? It's a transplant!* But I think that the word "transplant" is something that many people don't fully comprehend. *"Think about this! It's amazing! My heart was dead — I should have been dead. But instead, they took the heart of another person whose brain was dead and whose heart they had kept alive. And they took out my broken heart, and put in this new one. How incredible is that? In 1950 or 1960 or 1970, they couldn't do that! Think about how amazing that is. Think about the love of the donor family, allowing their loved one to live on inside of someone else's body — and what the recipient goes through. It's not just surgery. It's a miracle!"* His eyes had teared up as he spoke to me. He wanted to tell his friends how he felt, but he realized that no one was really listening. Again. He felt abandoned by his friends and co-workers. When he tried to reach out, he was cut off. "My wife and I went from being an influential couple to nothing. It was a cataclysmic change. I still struggle with it." He stopped trying to reach out and talk about it.

"You are alone when you are ill," he tells me.

So much of this story breaks my heart. I wonder if Anurag could see that his heart was broken. Perhaps even the first heart he got wasn't going to work, because his recovery was so filled with sadness. How could the new heart survive? The understanding that he no longer had the friends or community he thought he had was breaking him all over again. "The lessons I learned in India were missing. The camaraderie is what I miss most."

In 2015, Anurag had an antibody-mediated rejection, which, after almost two years, was unusual. But I do believe that the human condition can stump the medical community at any turn. As brilliant as these doctors and scientists are, no one can explain why the power of prayer or the resolve of the spirit can turn a certain death into a simple stepping stone in someone's life. For Anurag, his immunological response to the heart began to turn. The heart became very stiff and then his kidneys began to shut down. He endured between fifty and sixty biopsies. A hepatologist told him his liver was beginning to fail and his gallbladder was removed. "When I needed human touch the most, it was nowhere to be found." The heart got so big that it pressed against his lungs. Once again, he needed a new heart.

Finally, in July of 2020, Anurag got his second heart transplant, as well as a kidney transplant. He had a hernia on his sternum that was so big, that he couldn't wear a shirt. And one week after the transplant, he got a clot in his heart and they had to cut into his sternum again. But what happened next, was that he found people who wanted to help and who wanted to see him heal. His doctors at Cedars Sinai, and Doctor Deng at UCLA, along with Ava, were pulling for him and wanting him to heal. "It takes a community to heal a person, just like it takes a village to raise one," he tells me. Of course, Manuela has always been there. I get a glimpse of her, from time to time. A lovely little woman, patiently sitting with him. Loving him, correcting his timeline when necessary, and folding laundry while we talked for hours on a video chat. Sometimes, I'm sure; she was his whole village. "She wants to go to the Promised Land — to Jerusalem. So I am determined to take her there. And my daughter, Michelle, wants to take me rock climbing, so I am going to try that too."

Anurag is such a profound human being, I could never imagine anyone disregarding him or not acknowledging his ingenuity and wisdom. Quantum mechanics look at all Life from the atomic level. Not so much as one may have learned in physics class. But *Life* — from its smallest particle, growing into trees, flowers, people. And into a heart that lived, loved and lost inside of one human being, then placed into another, where it beats on. Where, in that, is the color of a man's skin? Perhaps a heart can break more than once, and perhaps stresses, if you don't find a way to deal with them, will keep teaching you the same lesson until you get it. And perhaps part of being brilliant is to understand that sometimes you have to stop and say the simple things to those closest to you. Sometimes, the simplest things are the most complicated to do.

"My son, Sean, is a distance cyclist," he tells me. "He can ride his bike for 100 miles. I cannot ride 100 miles, but I would like to ride just ten with him."

Anurag Saksena

Two-Time Heart and Kidney Transplant Recipient

Living with Manuela, Building a community, and

Getting ready for the ten-mile bike ride of his life.

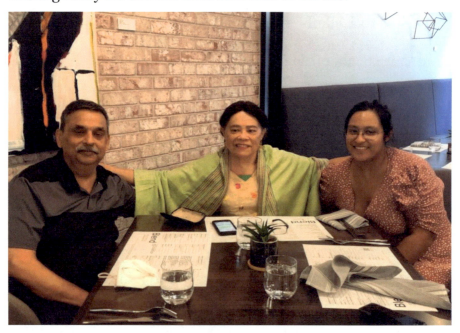

Anurag, Manuela and Michelle

CHAPTER NINETEEN

AVA'S HEART - FILLING AN EMPTY SPOT

Ava:

Heal. What a word! Where does one really even begin? I felt like I had already been through a lifetime of recovery. I still went to the hospital to do rehabilitation for my new heart, and what I really needed was to get rid of the walker. It was an anomaly to the dancer in my head. It was like being in a perpetual barre class and never getting to perform. And I needed to figure out how to correct how this interruption had affected Jade's life. This was such uncharted territory for me. I had no control. Jade was still a little girl. We had been the two musketeers for so long, that it was almost as if I'd broken a trust. I had unintentionally abandoned her and now, how could I expect her to jump back into life? Or go back to school? Would her little friends still take her in and be supportive? Every safety net I had carefully crafted had been cut, along with both of my parachutes. This was one fucked up free fall!

When I went to my rehab, I imagined dancing in my head, just to be able to get through it. I knew how to deal with physical pain, so I focused on that, because it was so much more tangible to me than the mental and emotional pain. I struck up conversations with other people there, and loved talking with my transplant coordinator, Jenna. She was positive and full of hope for every single patient she worked with. I watched her comfort the patients and their families. I could see people were scared. I never really had that, because I was already dead when they brought me in — but there it was! A space for me. Waiting for my physical therapist one day, I struck up a conversation with a family who was waiting to hear how their father/husband was after his heart transplant. I felt compelled to tell them my story because I was finally off the walker and getting ready to start pilates again. I saw their fear turn to hope — and then to gratitude for my words.

That was it. I had found a way to give back. I could be an advocate for the families of transplant patients — and the stronger I got, the better it made them feel. I could tell my story, and show them pictures of me ballroom dancing. They were comforted and hopeful. It felt amazing. I began to see the purpose emerge from my conversations. I applied to Cedars Sinai as a volunteer, so I could really help these families. Jenna directed me to patients I could visit in the hospital. I then became a part of the heart clinic, where patients who are potential recipients get evaluated. I was added to the list of people for those patients to meet with. With Jenna's help, I advocated for the importance of potential transplant recipients being given a picture of seeing the other side. I was there to offer hope. But the hospital needed to realize it too.

Obamacare enabled everyone to be able to get a transplant. But, I learned that housing and medications were a completely different story. There are states in our country where there are no transplant centers, which means that many transplant recipients must travel far from home to receive their heart or whatever they need. The "rules and regulations" say that you have to have nearby pre and post-transplant housing, or you cannot get an organ. People come from all around the country to Cedars Sinai and UCLA to get their transplants done — but they must have a place to live. The cost of three months of housing in a neighborhood near Cedars Sinai or UCLA Hospitals is prohibitive, to say the least. They are in a life or death situation without any resources. On top of that, post-transplant medication comes at a considerable cost. If the patient can't cover those costs, that too, means no transplant. When Jenna told me about a couple who worked to help transplant patients with their medication, I realized that my purpose was so much bigger than just talking with patients. I needed to find a way to help them with their housing and medication needs. I went straight to Cedars Sinai — right to the top of the food chain. I asked for assistance in setting transplant patients up with housing, and to this day, I will never forget the response:

"We are not in the hotel business."

While I understand that hospitals are a business and if making money is your only priority, then, of course that is the answer to my proposal. No, Cedars Sinai is not in the hotel business. But there is right — and there is wrong. People were dying — and I could see a way to help them live. But I wasn't going to get any help from this place. The truth about Cedars is, that they never supported me. I would venture to say that they even worked against me. Yes, they approved me for a heart, but I was an experiment. No one thought I was going to live, because they had never seen my illness attack a heart before. I was an anomaly, and they gave it a shot to see what would happen. And besides, I had great insurance.

Well, they didn't know who they were dealing with.

My friend, Rafi, told me to check out Change A Life Foundation. Her father started the foundation. During World War II, his family had hidden him in a Christian Blind School. After the war, his entire family except for one brother had were killed in the camps. Together, they came to the United States and started a business. He had never forgotten how he had been given a chance and he wanted to give back. He and his friend Lisa set up the Change A Life Foundation, where one could apply for a one-time grant to save someone's life. I asked to partner with them in my mission. Each patient who needed post-transplant housing and medication could apply for a grant, and I could help them do it. I was still recovering myself and every little step forward was a milestone in my unprecedented journey. Every misstep made me put my nose to the grindstone and push harder. And in perfect step with my newfound angels, I could make changes in the lives of these other patients. Once I realized this, it was like magic! The ability to help each patient coincided with my own recovery. A grand step matched a grand step. Here I was, dancing again!

I kept on with the Change A Life Foundation for about seven years, until Rafi's father died, and the foundation closed. By then, I had started Ava's Heart, through which I helped many families get $7500 grants for their post-transplant needs. I was introduced to One Legacy CEO, Tom Mone, with whom I partnered as well. One Legacy saves lives through organ, eye and tissue donation, and they also partner with Donate Life. I had met all of the right people for my cause, and as I grew stronger, I looked for a hospital partner that was more in step with what I was trying to accomplish. I had changed my care to UCLA — and a whole new world opened up. It was a world of acceptance of who I was and a world that had respect for what I was trying to accomplish. And it was a world where they wanted to help me. Being a creative thinker, I tried all kinds of ways to raise money for my own foundation. Sometimes it felt a bit like high school car washing fundraisers, until I came up with my gala event: Ava's Heart Hero's Ball. It is an annual fundraising event, where there is a dinner, entertainment, and an auction. It raises awareness within and about organ transplantation, honoring doctors, transplant donors and recipients, celebrities and anyone else who has made significant contributions to the transplant community.

Families who are in need of a transplant, or who are donating organs contact me online and let me know what they need. I get on the phone with them because I always want them to know that there is a real person on the other end of the online form. Understanding what these families are dealing with requires human contact. I would like to take my business to a national level, but there is a lack of desire to merge similar organizations. I don't know if that's ego-driven, or if it comes from a lack of wanting to take a leap of faith, but I have always believed that there is strength in numbers. And I have always believed that if I was singing in a choir, our collective voices would be so much more powerful than mine alone.

CHAPTER TWENTY
BETHANY AND HANNAH KEIME -
ACTIVISTS, INFLUENCERS FOR HCM

I am writing this book in the time of Covid, and as much as I don't like to shop online because I can't touch everything, I similarly don't like to interview people without seeing them. When the video interview opened, there were two beautiful, young ladies smiling back at me. Of course, I took the traditional "they don't look sick at all" approach to the interview.

And I was right.

As I ask them about their stories — the same but different — Hannah is the first to start talking. Often moving in and out of the picture, she is a tall, pretty brunette, who is smiling and talking as she shifts around. Hannah is funny. She has a captivating sense of humor, even when she tells me about the first time the doctor told her she was going to need a defibrillator and then at some point, a heart transplant.

Hannah used to dance and play basketball. She is the eighth of nine children and clearly holds her own — well — dominates a conversation.

When she was 17, she fainted at her brother's 14th birthday party — which, years later and getting ready for college, she says, he is still not pleased with. After her diagnosis, on April 10, 2015, Hannah had her defibrillator implanted. She said that the transplant had been brought up several times saying, "I know down the line I will probably need a heart". Hannah is twenty-one years old, as is my eldest daughter, also an athlete. She is tall and slender, funny and vivacious. Hannah made the decision to quit basketball and dance (sort of). She was told that shuffleboard and golf were okay, but instead, Hannah turned to theatrical dance/movement and acting. That doesn't exactly seem like a 'shuffleboard" to me. Six months after it was implanted, her defibrillator did its job. At 3:30am, when her heart rate went up to 253 beats per minute, she went unconscious. Had she not had the implant, she would never have awakened. I stare at this extraordinary young woman, smiling and chatting through her story:

"And then, two years later, I got shocked again! I was in a staged dancing battle with my best friend, and you know what it felt like? I mean, I thought She hit me in the chest! It was like a sledgehammer that hit a home run!"

She thought it was her friend hitting her in the dance battle with such force, that it threw her head back. It wasn't until she spoke to her doctor later, that she found out the defibrillator, once again, was doing its job, only this time, she was awake — on stage — dancing.

I ask about faith, because it is a constant with everyone I have spoken to along this journey. Hannah begins to say, "In the Spoken Word we say . . ." when Bethany taps her headphone and we get cut off. They are sharing air pods — Bethany sitting in a chair, with Hannah teetering on the arm precariously. I think about when my sister and I tried to squeeze both of our heads into the Bose headphones in 1974, so we could listen to Ruby Tuesday together.

Sisters.

We get reconnected.

Hannah says she owes her life to Jesus Christ, and so she took some time off school to go on an 18-month mission. Her eyes sparkle as she talks about the "cool and exotic" places she was supposed to travel to all over the world. But the Church saw things a little differently. They didn't want her to be somewhere outside of the United States, should anything go awry with her heart, so they sent her to Salt Lake City in Temple Square. She met people from all over the world — cool and exotic places — and taught them about "who we are". She was then called to serve in Twin Falls, Idaho, where she taught English to people from The Democratic Republic of Congo. "They were very cool and exotic people," she says, laughing.

This was all by the age of twenty-one, knowing that she could have died twice, had it not been for her implanted defibrillator, knowing that she will one day need a heart transplant.

"Me and God both know I can serve," she tells me.

Bethany sits quietly beside her sister, smiling as she tells her story and laughing when Hannah is joking around. She is number seven of nine children, and had her defibrillator implanted on January 29, 2018. She had passed out twice, and went to the doctor praying with every ounce of her breath that she would not also need the defibrillator like her sister. But she did. "It's crushing to be told you can't do what you love", she says. I think about the dance studio where I trained so long ago. I wasn't your typical dancer. I was really strong and I didn't even look the part. But in every single studio, there were posters: *If you can dream it, you can do it!* — or — *Never give up on something you really want. It's difficult to wait, but it's more difficult to regret.* Those things kept me going because dance was never just about the movement. Dancing sets your spirit free. It makes you feel like you are beautiful, even if that isn't how you see yourself. And sometimes it feels like the music was written just for that very moment, whatever that moment may be. It's perfect and it's different for everyone — so when someone says to you, "You have to stop . . ."

Well . . . sometimes you just can't.

"We are truly blessed," Bethany says. "God has given this to us because He knows we can handle it." At first glance, her Instagram page is filled with images of her, like any other young woman her age. But then you take a closer look. You watch the videos and you read the decorated posts. A sexy bathing suit pose, as she pulls herself from the water, glancing back toward the camera. Take a closer look and you can see the outline of her implanted defibrillator along her side, under her skin. There's a video titled "The Bionic Woman", where she shows a creative rendition of the procedure for the implant. It shows her exercising and even dancing on pointe. It screams at the viewer: "I can do everything I could do before! I am strong and beautiful!" Bethany bears a slight resemblance to Kate Beckinsale, so it floors me to hear her say that she struggles with her appearance. I think about my years as a dancer. I understand, but as a much older woman now, I want her to know how incredible she is. I watch a video of her dancing and I can see her spirit is so free. She is breathtaking,

Their Instagram page is titled Heartcharged. It is maintained and posted on by both sisters, along with their mother, Stephanie. I think Stephanie must be an amazing woman. Mother of nine children. They both describe her as their biggest advocate, super smart, a woman who has dedicated her life to them and who encourages them to always follow their dreams . . . And there's that dance studio poster again: *Follow Your Dreams*

The page and the Keime sisters, with their implanted defibrillators, are seeking to make it part of every pediatric physical to check for the gene mutation that causes Hypertrophic Cardiomyopathy. They are trying to make it mandatory through federal legislation. Their aunt has it, so their mother got checked, and she also has it. Their aunt needed a valve replacement, while their mother is still okay. Out of the nine children only Bethany and Hannah have it. They have more severe cases than their mother or their aunt, and had to have the implants. "It's the leading cause of deaths of young athletes on the court or on the field," Hannah tells me. I looked that up, and it is, in fact, accurate.

After my call with the Keime sisters, I can't stop thinking about how strong and positive they both are. I left that call feeling uplifted and hopeful . . . just because of them. I think back to the part of the conversation when Hannah had been cut off: "In the Spoken Word, we say —"

I look that up on the internet, and here's what I found:

> *Words are singularly the most powerful force available to Humanity.*
>
> *God's words have Life — They bring Life*

Here are these two bright spirits in the world — knowing one or both of them will likely one day need a heart transplant — joyfully speaking about their lives and trying to make the knowledge of Hypertrophic Cardiomyopathy a mandated test for all kids. Teaching English to people seeking a better life and living by the perfect example of bravery, beauty, and strength.

Go Change the World, Ladies!

Bethany and Hannah Keime

Activists, Living with HCM

Leading By Example, Every Day

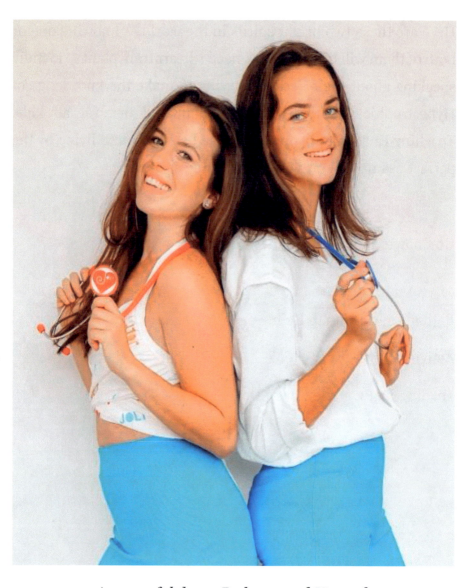

A powerful duo – Bethany and Hannah

CHAPTER TWENTY-ONE
JESSICA OSTRAND - IT IS WHAT IT IS

Jessica is the youngest of three children, born to Stephanie and Jeremy Ostrand at Denver Children's Hospital. They are the kind of couple who have been together for so long and been through so much, that they finish each other's sentences. And yet remain decidedly different. Stephanie is pragmatic. She re-educates herself for whatever situation she is in. She learns on the fly and takes everything in stride. Jeremy speaks poignantly about his family, relating more to the emotional side of their journey together. Twenty weeks into her pregnancy with Jessica, they knew she was going to have to have heart surgery. She had coarctation of the aorta and atrioventricular canal defects. So Jessica had her first heart surgery when she was only 4 days old. Looking back at me from the interview screen is a family who is living both in the middle of, and on the other side of a veritable procession of medical roadblocks in their lives. It's something many of us hear about, but cannot, or perhaps don't ever bother, to imagine what that would be like. Stephanie had atrioventricular canal issues and had repairs done to her own heart when she was just 26 years old. She was a young mother then, with two little boys at home. The eldest, Jonathan, who is now 25, had his first surgery when he was only one year old. He has Pulmonary Stenosis. That means that the valve that pumps blood from the heart to the lungs is too small, or too narrow or too stiff, so it cannot let the blood out sufficiently to send it to the lungs. So the heart has to work harder, causing thickening of the right ventricle (one of the four chambers of the heart) and strains the heart. It is congenital, and has nothing to do with anything the mother did or didn't do. At 15 years old, when Jonathon was running to class, his heart stopped. His friends did CPR on him until an ambulance arrived, and he had an AICD (Automatic Implantable Cardioverter Defibrillator) implanted, and had a pulmonary valve replaced. An AICD is a combination pacemaker and defibrillator, Jeremy explains to me. I am furiously taking notes. I look back to the screen and see Stephanie, Jeremy and Jessica looking at me quizzically. This interview is for Jessica. Of their three children, only Joseph, their middle child, is free of cardiovascular issues — but not wanting to be left out of the procession, he was born at only 27 weeks, due to placenta previa.

At five months old, Jessica got her first heart transplant. She had been considered an FTT infant (failure to thrive) due to lack of weight gain. She had a hypoplastic left heart, which includes underdevelopment of the left ventricle and ascending aorta, underdevelopment of the aortic and mitral valves, narrowing of the aorta, atrial septal defect (hole in the wall of the upper chambers of the heart), and PDA, or patent ductus arteriosus, which, if left open, can lead to cardiac shock and death.

I listed everything there, as evidence that the hope that anything else could have been done for this little fighter was put to rest. She needed a transplant and she got one, but Stephanie and Jeremy were also told that Jessica would eventually need another heart. And by the age of 4, the rejection had begun. She was vomiting every day and had to have an NG tube inserted, a tube that is inserted through the nose, down through the esophagus and into the stomach. Everything caused her to have chest pains. Stephanie would change the tube every week. She was a preschool teacher at the time. Their transplant coordinator encouraged Stephanie to become a nurse. And she did. She has a paralegal license, and a CNA license, and is looking forward to getting a BNA. She now works at RADI Children's Hospital in San Diego. By the age of 8, Jessica was getting mouth sores because her anti-rejection meds were off. The family, who had relocated to Temecula, drove up to UCLA for Jessica's second heart transplant. That's where they met Ava.

Jeremy's eyes tear up when I ask him about Ava. "Ava is God's gift, "he says. His voice falters slightly. "She brings love. She brings everything. I would do anything for that woman."

I find it stunning that this family, who has been through so much, finds time to see the beauty in other people. It's a genuine love and affection for someone, and an understanding of the magnitude of Ava's work and of the purity in her heart. And for all of their own suffering, they can still see that in another person.

Jessica is a pretty, slightly serious 16-year-old girl with long, straight hair and round glasses. Like any teenager, she rolls her eyes a little when her parents say something embarrassing. Anything. Her resilience flies off the screen. It has been eight years since her second heart transplant, and she plays basketball and runs track — hurdles, actually. If you have ever tried hurdles, you know how much more work it is. But she loves it, and apparently, her newest heart is fine with it. She has also been on the swim team and made the cheerleading squad. Amazingly, the roadblocks she encountered after the second heart transplant were not because of the transplant itself but because of callous and insensitive teachers in school. Shortly after her transplant, in the *third grade*, a teacher mocked her for always needing to sit down and rest "just when things got a little tougher on the playground". Jessica's grandmother was on the playground with her. She explained to the cold-hearted educator that Jessica had developed Osteopenia (the loss of bone mass), as a result of taking the anti-rejections medication. Another time, during a classroom experiment, a teacher would not let Jessica participate because it required her to hold her breath underwater for 30 seconds, announcing to the entire class that "Jessica's heart might explode". What unimaginable cruelty not to do everything in their power to learn about what was needed to support their young student. I would think they would want to be as educated as possible. "My coaches are different," Jessica tells me. "They trust me to explain how I am feeling. I appreciate that trust." She has a direct way of delivering her words, and I wish she had told her teacher how ignorant his comments about her heart exploding were. I am quite sure he would never have said such a thing to any student ever again.

During her pregnancy with Jessica, Stephanie developed gestational diabetes, and has since developed type II diabetes, so on top of everything else, she struggles with a laundry list of medications needed for herself and two of her children. But here they are, squished together on a sofa in front of their computer screen, talking graciously to me. When I ask them how they do it, Jeremy smiles slightly. "Our motto is, *It is what it is*. We leave our jobs. We talk to the Lord every day. And, when it comes to the health of our kids, we show up." He recalls when they were told in 2013 that they'd found a heart for Jessica. "I was on the balcony, "he says, "watching her play with a remote control mustang." That is a picture emblazoned into his mind. Such a normal scene. But with unimaginable heartache associated with it. Although it must have been such a relief that a heart had become available, the flip side of that is equally overwhelming. Wherever the heart came from, it was a gift from God and from the donor family.

She's a normal kid with an extraordinary story and a resolve that rivals the greatest of humanity. She had wanted to be in the military but learned that she would be turned down due to her health issues. So what next? "A doctor or a lawyer, "she says, confidently, "and I want to move back to Colorado. I miss it".

Personally, I would be honored to have her serve my country, be my doctor or my lawyer, or whatever she chooses to become. There is not a doubt in my mind that she will achieve it.

Jessica Ostrand lives in Temecula, California.

She is a fighter.

And she will be the best at whatever she chooses to do.

I can feel it.

Double Heart Transplant Recipient

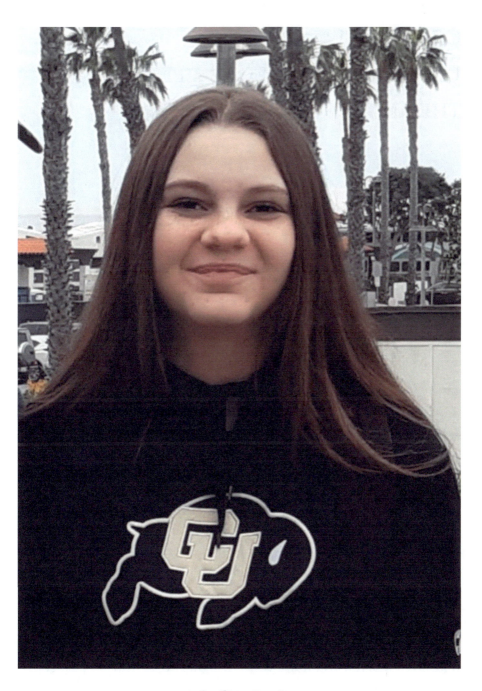

A Smiling Jessica

CHAPTER TWENTY-TWO
LILLY AND FELIX LEON - A FEATHER FOR THE ANGEL

"I'm in shock," Lilly tells me. "I'm starting to feel it now though." She is gorgeous and looks like she could be 18 or 19 years old, but she is standing with a four-month-old infant . . . and she tells me she has a three-year-old . . . and a nine-year-old. She has enormous brown eyes and dark brown hair, and she is hugging her newest child, Dylan, close to her chest. When I ask her about her brother, Felix, an instant of sadness washes over her face. It's difficult to distinguish what it means. Desperation for answers or a lack of understanding about the whirlwind that whipped through the Leon family in the preceding months. But I think it was a sort of breathless sorrow. The kind where you are left questioning God, and the kind where you wake up day after day, hoping that it was all a terrible nightmare. But the thing that made you sad is still there.

Lilly was already ten years old when Felix was born on May 30, 1999, so she had to watch him a lot. Her initial impression of him was, "Well, he had a ton of energy!" I laughed to myself. My eldest daughter was ten when my youngest was born, and we also relied on her to babysit. Then Lilly smiles. "And he loved Hot Wheels!" And there it was again: little boys and their toy cars. But Felix was different. "It was always the four of us," Lilly says, as the sadness washes over her again. She tells me how Felix used to ask his parents for cast-off clothing that no one wanted. On his own, he would gather up a bag, buy some large pizzas, and distribute clothing and food to the homeless people in their Compton neighborhood. For a teenage boy, for anyone, really, it was such a selfless gesture. To keep himself looking fit, he rode his bike everywhere. And every single day, without fail, he rode from Compton to Carson, to visit with his favorite priest at his favorite church. He was so close to God, that his priest later told Lilly, "I felt that maybe he asked God to take him. He was the kindest, most giving person I've ever met."

Lilly struggles with our conversation. Felix had only been gone a little less than three months. It didn't seem real to her. Her own baby had been born only five weeks before Felix had died, and the rise and fall of emotions must have taken quite a toll.

"In April, she said, he was fine — at the beginning. He went to Compton College. He was a great student. He never took any pills for anything. Not aspirin or ibuprofen. Nothing. But for some reason, he decided he wanted to take the supplement biotin. He took a 10,000 mcg dose, which, according to most websites, is within the normal range. The following day, he had terrible stomach pains. They got so bad, that he went to the emergency room in the late afternoon. He was released at 1:30 am the following morning, and went home, where he lived with his parents. He was only twenty-one years old and the hospital had determined that it was likely some kind of an allergic reaction.

But when Lilly stopped by the following day to check up on him, he showed her his legs, which were completely swollen. She told him to return to the ER, but because Covid was rampant in early April 2020, they wouldn't admit him. Instead, he had a video chat with a doctor, who told him not to worry, and that he would eventually "pee it all out". Another day passed, and he has rushed to the ER again. His swelling had increased and later turned out to be brain swelling. He was immediately taken into surgery. The family was informed that Felix's brain swelling was due to Thrombosis, leading to a massive stroke. He was intubated. When he woke up from surgery, he was told that he had lost most functions on the right side of his body. After two months in the hospital and an acute rehabilitation facility, he was finally discharged and sent home.

I was shocked at the fact that Felix had been sent home after his very first hospital visit. Even from my limited research I am aware that biotin can cause stomach upset, and allergic reactions, including swelling of the legs, throat and face. And it can also lead to dangerously low blood sugar, causing insulin to react by raising the blood sugar level to the point that it can cause a blood clot or stroke. It can skew blood work, notably that of cardiac troponins, which are markers used to diagnose a heart attack. But, he was only twenty-one. Not even seasoned medical professionals usually associate any swelling with heart attacks or strokes at such a young age.

In doing his therapy from home, the nurse noted that his blood pressure was extremely low, as was his heart rate. Athletic people do have lower blood pressure. But at that point, Felix was diagnosed with congestive heart failure. They were to medicate him for congestive heart failure, until he displayed signs of a viral infection. That, too, turned out to be another allergic reaction to the medications he was taking. They then determined, at 21-years-old, that Felix was going to need a heart transplant. It was June. Just two months before, this loving young man had been riding his bike to church every single day, feeding the homeless, having sandwich lunches with his mom, and playing with his little nieces, Jayleen and Delaney. They called him "Juju".

Doctors at Cedars Sinai determined that they would insert a PICC line and that he would be listed for a heart transplant. A nurse came to the house and inserted the PICC line and put on a gauze sleeve. Lilly described the gauze sleeve to me carefully, like it was the last thing she remembered about him.

A rash developed around the PICC line, and Felix was again taken to Cedars. Again, because of Covid's restrictions, his parents and his sister had to say goodbye to him at the door. Felix was still struggling to regain his speech, so the family watched him, until he was gone from sight without a verbal goodbye from him. That night in the hospital, Felix's heart was pumping so slowly, that they thought that they would have to install a pump, but had to opt for an ECMO machine instead while he waited for a heart. At midnight, Felix began to bleed, and again, the doctors had to surgically stabilize him. By midnight, he did stabilize, and the following day, they got a heart. The surgery was successful, and the hospital called Felix's parents and Lilly to tell them that they would be waking him up the following day.

But Felix was never to wake up.

That night, The hospital again called the Leon family to tell them that Felix had suffered another massive stroke — this time on the left side of his brain.

"We held on to God and we prayed for a miracle," Lilly told me, through tears. "They officially declared him brain dead three days later."

Maybe the miracle *was Felix*. And maybe God wanted him to come home, because that was where he belonged.

His parents were approached immediately, as it has to be, to become a donor, and of course, they knew Felix would have wanted that. So on the day he died, Felix donated his new heart, his kidneys, liver, eyes and bone marrow.

That's when Ava came in. The families of organ donors don't always have a means of burial or cremation. One Legacy referred Lilly to Ava, for help with Felix's cremation. He had saved at least five lives that day. Ava quietly listened to Lilly's story. And then she made the call to cover his cremation.

Somehow, being a donor didn't give Lilly much comfort. I asked her if she had someone to talk to and how her kids were doing.

Then I asked her about her dreams. She told me that both she and her mother had dreams, but that when they woke up, neither of them could remember them. So I asked about the kids. And she lit up. "Yes!" She said, "They dream about him, and they remember their dreams!" Jayleen, who is nine, was up early in Grandma's living room one morning, holding a picture of Felix. She knew Uncle Felix had gone to Heaven before anyone told her. She said, "He told me he is working and he is happy. And tell Nana to stop crying." And little Delaney dreamt that she was in a white park, with a white playground and white trees, and she told Lilly, "Juju will always be with us."

"Was there anything else?" I ask. Lilly is now smiling as she thinks about what her girls were dreaming about.

"Yes," she says. "It's the strangest thing . . ."

Shortly after Felix passed, his mother found a bright green feather in the middle of her living room floor. She thought back to when he had asked her if she believed in reincarnation because if it was real, he wanted to come back as a bird.

They continue to find feathers in the strangest places — a large white one on the bed where he slept, and another on the factory floor where his father works. So they are collecting them.

After all, an angel needs his wings.

Lilly and Felix Leon,

A sister and brother separated on earth,

Visiting in their dreams of white playgrounds,

With green hummingbirds and parrots.

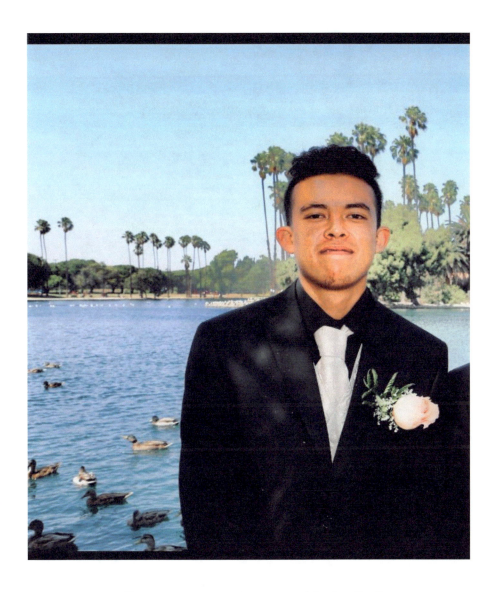

Felix Leon – Hanging out with the ducks

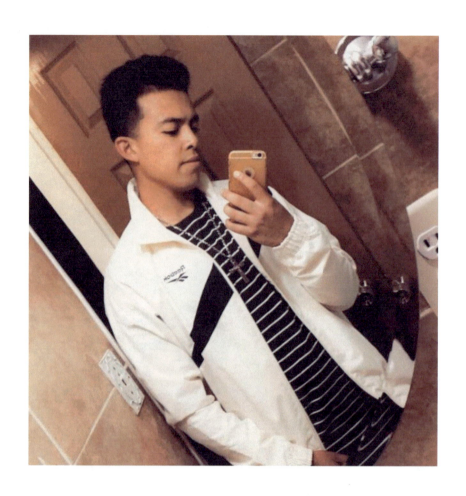

Felix just being a kid

CHAPTER TWENTY-THREE
THE ONE THING THAT COULD BREAK MY HEART AGAIN

Sometimes, when things get too tough to handle, even the strongest of us have to stuff our feelings down to get through it. Ava did that.

There wasn't anyone there from her family to make her meals, or to encourage her to keep moving forward. There were times when she wanted to give up, but the dancer and the mom inside of her wouldn't let that happen. She often waited for a call from her sister or her brother to say, "Hey! I'm here, but if you need me to come closer, I can." She knew that in writing this book, things were going to boil to the surface.

And they did.

By the end of September 2020, Ava had read through everything we had written together several times.

Ava:

It was hard to read a lot of this, because of the truth of what happened. Every day that passed, I would pick it up and read a little more. I suppose I had to run away from it a bit in order to survive. I have spent many, many days trying to help people navigate through their transplant journeys. I have listened to donor families and helped wherever I could, and it has been heartbreaking and fulfilling in equal measure. But seeing all of the families coming together for one another. Watching friends come in and help. Getting letters of appreciation from patients and their families and from people who have lost their loved ones. That still leaves a massive hole in my life. I have to protect my own heart with ferocity because it hurts so desperately not to be able to say what I need to say to my own family. And the feeling that it was all so unnecessary produces growing anger that I have had to let go of. It's difficult, though, when you realize that most of the people in your family would have preferred for you to have passed on, so they wouldn't have to deal with the person you became down the line. The stronger, better, more amazing person.

As I read the written words, I needed to find sympathy for Michael, who had so much anger toward me. He was hateful. I needed to find forgiveness for people who at some point or another, and for their own reasons, could not be there for me. I needed to find a way to let go of some of my friends when I realized that they were going to be detrimental to my continued recovery. Those friends who I had known, loved, laughed and cried with for thirty or more years. Maybe it was just getting older, or maybe I didn't pay close enough attention before I got sick, but I could no longer allow the negativity to poison me and my new heart. Someone died to give me this heart, and I am bound to protect it with every ounce of my being until it ceases to beat in my chest.

I am writing this, because the journey of life, love, recovery, helping people, and becoming part of a community I could not have imagined pre-2009, is an imperfect journey. There are still struggles. There are still money problems and frustrations over relationships, and there is still stress . . . Life still gets in the way. And it will for everyone. We can be thankful for everything we have been given, for our donors and for our second and third chances. But when we walk down the street, no one we pass will know what we have endured. No one will know that we carry another human being inside of us, that the little things that change about us after our transplants, might be from our donors. We are the living symbols of the truest form of spirituality and connection to everyone and everything in the universe.

I have spoken to so many transplant recipients and donor families along this journey, and I marvel at the ability people have to live always looking forward. It is such a gift, because looking back is destructive. We all have regrets. It's only human. So many people say they don't believe in regrets, but the real trick is not to live in them. My journey has been one of patience. Learning to take one moment at a time, then one day at a time, while never wishing away a single one of those days. The poison of regret is the one thing that could break my heart again.

And so, my personal journey of forgiveness continues.

As for the transplant journey, I have found that the dictionary gives all answers to even the most difficult questions, simply by defining what words really mean, in their most literal format. In a pamphlet I wrote, I looked upon my changing attitudes as chapters, like *Fear to Courage*. According to verywellmind.com, Fear is a primitive, natural and powerful human emotion. It involves a universal biochemical response as well as a high individual emotional response. Fear alerts us to the presence of danger or the threat of harm, whether that danger is physical or psychological. According to Webster's Dictionary, Fear is a reason for dread or apprehension. Any and all of these so perfectly describe how someone feels, when trying to grasp the concept that they need an organ transplant. You are the one, alone, who is waiting for someone else to die, so that you can have a new life. It is highly individual — wanting to stay alive is primitive — waiting for the death of another human being crosses deep psychological boundaries. I was already dead when this decision was made for me, but in dealing with transplant recipients and donor families, I have shared their deepest fears and tried to help them to navigate the darker emotions associated with organ transplants. Life happens, and you can't stop it or stall it — but you *can* listen to people when they need to talk about how they are feeling — and you *can* let them know that they are not alone. When recipients are told, "We found you a heart!", they all know that it wasn't discarded by the side of the road, and they are quietly cognisant of the fact that another life has just been lost, and that, while we sigh a breath of relief, somewhere there is a family filled with grief. It seems somehow fitting that those two emotions rhyme.

Courage is defined as the mental or moral strength to venture, persevere, and withstand danger, fear, or difficulty. It is even defined as "to persevere *without* fear", which I find impossible, because without fear, there could be no courage. There are different types of courage, though, and courage begins with moral courage. Moral courage comes with the struggle, and then the acceptance that because someone else died, I was given a second chance at life. The intellectual courage comes from understanding that the process of an organ transplant is a medical miracle. Someone must be kept alive while their brain no longer functions, so that their organs may be moved to another person's body. That person's brain is still alive but has lost the function of one or more organs. That in itself is a testament to the universal connection that branches into the metaphysical sense of reality — at least for many of us. It's not just "an operation". It's an exchange of one life for another, in some sense of universal understanding. And then there is disciplined courage, where you choose to go forward with the transplant, knowing all of these things. And you find the strength to trust in the miracle and persevere with whatever is going to come next. You live in the hope that the transplant will work, and you believe with every sense of your being, that your body will not let you down and reject the gift.

Fear turns to courage.

And then there's the wait. You are in this alone. You wait for an organ. You wait to wake up. You wait for the pain to stop. You wait in the hope of no rejection. So what is the definition of waiting? Waiting means to remain stationary in readiness or expectation, to look forward expectantly, or to hold back expectantly. It is fascinating that this definition describes more the attitude of the one who waits. Are you someone who looks forward expectantly? Or are you someone who holds back expectantly? For me, I was waiting to be able to move. Waiting to be able to speak. Waiting for someone, — *anyone* — to walk into my room. I waited for my uncle to become more human and I waited for my sister to tell me "Please don't die on me Ava! Remember who we used to be?" I waited for the doctor to come to tell me my body was rejecting the heart and I waited for something to wet my lips, scratch my nose, or turn on my TV. I waited for the sounds of Fernando's footsteps in the hallway, hoping he would pass me by. I waited for the chance to dance again, and I waited for my daughter's little hand in mine.

I waited for every fucking second to tick by, so I could start the next minute, and then I would count the seconds again.

According to Google Dictionary, patience is defined as the capacity to accept or tolerate delay, trouble or suffering without getting angry or upset. How a dictionary defines every attitude or situation of every person in fifteen words is magical. And that was it. The acceptance of suffering gives freedom from the agony of the wait. There I was, unable to move or speak. My mind could have taken me to a place where I would break, but instead, I leaned into a Higher Power. I spoke to God, and remembered the promise I made to Him. It helped me to have faith in something bigger than myself, and even in the moments today when I have to wait with other recipients, I can absorb some of their agonies by sharing my experience, praying for them, and keeping my faith always in the forefront. Faith will get you through the worst of days and it will help you find light in the darkest corners. And although, as I said, I am always careful not to wish time away, I can fill it with hope and faith in something better — not just for myself — but for every single person I meet along my journey. I think that people often focus on what they could have done to prevent their illness from taking over their lives. It's true that there are lessons in every step of our lives, but not finger-pointing lessons. Sometimes they are just to teach us how strong and resilient we are. I learned patience in the truest sense of the word. It wasn't something I had previously needed to dabble in, even though I had been through breast cancer, a mastectomy, and two hip replacements. My recovery had always been quick and my impatience had always worked in my favor. This time was different. So I accepted the waiting and I looked forward to the visits, the therapy, and set goals for myself that I looked forward to conquering. I prayed to God and kept my promise in the front of my mind. And somewhere along the way, I realized that the agony had subsided and the patience necessary to heal had set in.

Waiting turns to patience.

I suppose that, for me, there is still an elusive lesson for forgiveness when it comes to Saul and to other members of my family. I have a huge capacity to forgive, but for me, it has been the most difficult part of my journey when it comes to my family. I approach them with a heart that broke and had to be replaced, and they don't understand the enormity of that. I want to scream at them and shake them and cry, "Can't you hear me?? I have suffered so terribly!!" And in my most recent letter to some of them, one family member responded, "Ava, why do you keep writing us stuff like this?"

Because I wanted — I needed — someone to care.

But sometimes, you just have to give people back to the universe.

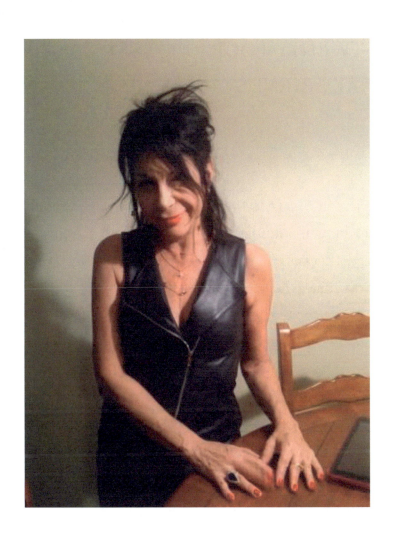

CHAPTER TWENTY-FOUR
MY ETERNAL FRIENDS

Ava:

There was one lesson I learned throughout my journey. Friends can be a fickle bunch. I understand how difficult a journey everything was — because I was in it. I had no choice. What surprised me was that, when the going got really tough, people disappeared. Anurag spoke about the people who would call and leave messages because they didn't want to actually hear how he was doing. There was no one to listen to this crazy notion that someone else's heart was beating inside of your body. The people who had been close and loving — who had been willing to share a bottle of wine and talk about business or about people, or about amazing new ideas . . . they had all gone. There was a new reality, a new heart and my same body that definitely didn't work the same as it used to.

But, as others dropped by the wayside, I knew that Clare and David would still be there.

By the time I left the hospital, Clare had come to take care of me and David was always present. Our beautiful home had been sold, so he was no longer my touchstone next door, but it was still the three of us, nevertheless, now in a little apartment, baking cookies in our dance leotards.

As I look around my writing table today, I am being helped by people who maybe are not mentioned in my book. Not because they are not true friends, but because throughout this journey, I find some old and some new friends. I have rekindled some relationships and have had to give others back to the universe. I used to think friends were forever, because I chose them. They were not forced on me. But friends can surprise you and even disappoint you. My transplant was a testament to that. But something beautiful happened too. It's funny how that works. The yin and the yang. Out of the disappearance of many of my friends, deeper, more meaningful relationships blossomed. I found people I could count on no matter how messy things got. They are my eternal flowers. And no matter where we all go in our lives from this moment on, these are the friends who will stand by with the strength and grace of what defines friendship.

CHAPTER TWENTY-FIVE
ENOUGH - (For David)

Enough

As the sun goes down

And the shadows grow long

And the dancing slows

To a slower song

Your light shines as brightly

On the day we first met

To me, you are eternal

A prince — and yet

Your silence is not lost

On my once deaf ears

Your absence fills my heart

With our lost hopes and fears

You will always be

My touchstone of all friends

My partner, my savior

Who never breaks, only bends

And if by chance there was a crack

And you have just grown tired

Know that somewhere in the world

You are deeply, truly admired

It's hard to say how you will land in the world

But in the thousands of days we would talk

That this I know in my heart of hearts

You carried me when I could not walk

For the rest of ever

There is no never

We only dance

To a setting sun

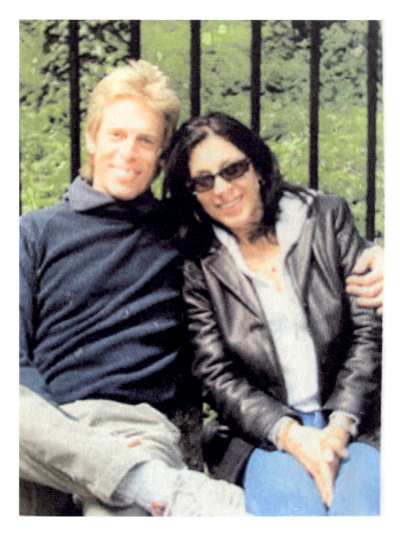

David and Ava

CHAPTER TWENTY-SIX
SIDRA FRANKLIN LOCURTO - SOUL SISTER

My video chat opened to a blonde lady in a hat, with giant, almost unreal eyes. When they say that the eyes are the windows to the soul, they must have been looking at Sidra.

Ava and Sidra met walking out of a dance class at a place called Swerve in Los Angeles. She was a volunteer at Cedars Sinai and used to bring her dog in as a therapy dog. It was two or three years after Ava's transplant, and they became immediate and intimate friends. And I can see why. Sidra is a singer, a painter, a dancer, a designer of interiors and landscapes, a make-up artist, an actress, a poet, a writer, a mom, a wife, a volunteer and an animal lover. Not necessarily in that order. She is also from Long Island, just like Clare. "I always saw my bigger life", she tells me. "I couldn't get out and move to New York City fast enough." She is from South Bellmore, between the canals and close to Jones Beach. In looking all of that up, I understand leaving. But not because it isn't beautiful. There is an amphitheater literally on the water, so that the backdrop of the stage is the ocean. It's incredible. But the Atlantic Ocean is something of an enigma to me. It is hauntingly desolate, mysterious and cold, and invokes feelings of intense sadness in me. At the same time, I could stand on the shore and watch the waves for the rest of my life and be perfectly happy. I always imagine it with tall grasses and sandy beaches, whereas I see the Pacific Ocean as being lined with palm trees, evergreens, and cliffs. I look around the area on Google Earth, and I find Amityville. Like . . . the house? Or like Jaws? It's a quiet enough place that I understand needing something else — especially for someone with Sidra's spirit. Her New York accent, though faint, slips out when she gets more excitedly talking. My Canadian accent comes out when I've had one too many glasses of wine.

By her own admission, Sidra walks to the beat of her own drum. She is outspoken and passionate. So she, of course, found a natural kinship with Ava. She moved to New York City when she was 18. There was an excitement there that didn't exist back home. There were so many different people and the cultural scene took her breath away. She dove in. She knew from the age of 8 that she was going to be there. Without question.

Without question. That's the phrase that best describes Sidra. When her other friend needed a second heart transplant, Sidra got a note that her friend had told the doctor that if she did not have a viable heart by a certain date, she wanted her defibrillator shut off. Sidra, without a moment of hesitation, told her friend, "No, you are not going to shut off your defibrillator. No, you are not going to stop fighting. No, you are not going to give up." Sometimes, the decisions we make are clearer to a friend who is looking in, because we can get in our own way, and make decisions based on fear or to eliminate pain. Sometimes a friend telling you to keep fighting is the only thing that gets you to the next day. That's Sidra. "I don't like it when she (Ava) gets down." I had to agree with her, but what struck me more than that, was the deep understanding that this woman has for her friend. She knows how much it takes for Ava to stop, even for a second. She seems never to feel overwhelmed by her own life, by the stories of the people who need her help, or by any of the everyday things that can make us pause for a moment or hesitate in our own stories. Even as I wrote these words, Ava had to turn down two donor families in need of assistance this morning. In the age of Covid, there are not many donations coming into Ava's Heart. "But the thing with Ava is, that every time she goes to the depths of despair, something amazing happens." That's true. But it never just happens, and even as she tells me this, we are both keenly aware that Ava's sense of never giving up is what makes amazing things happen. It's not magic. It's brutally hard, unforgiving work, and many people don't get the help they need and that chips away at her. Sidra knows that.

Her intuition is striking. She talks to me about things we have in common, like we are old friends, and yet, we have only met once in passing. "When Covid started," she tells me, "I felt like my powers of intuition were shut off." Creative people have that thing in common, where they see into the soul of whatever they are looking at. That's why we become so enamoured by a painting or a photograph, or by a beautiful dance, or a piece of music. Something about it hits us in the deepest part of ourselves, and we feel like the artist "gets" us. Sidra never knew any of the details about Ava's life with her sister, Mona, before the end of Mona's life. She didn't know that they were kindred spirits, and that Ava needed her sister always. But she filled the void that Mona left. Not in a way that Mona was replaceable. She wasn't. But going out into the world without Mona left a pain of unfulfilled conversations and unanswered questions. And although Sidra couldn't speak for Mona, she became a sister to Ava. When she talks to me about their conversations, she gets that in your face, New Yorker boldness and tells Ava how things are going to be. Everything is said with a blend of love and frankness, brutal honesty and compassion. "It's funny though. I feel older than Ava. We are kindred spirits — like sisters —, but she seems like she is only 18. That's why chronological age doesn't mean anything to me. Sometimes it just doesn't fit."

The conversation switches to her son, Wil. She speaks about her mother, and how she regrets not bringing her out to Los Angeles. "She ended up in a terrible place, and Wil is like me. He can tell things like that." She tells me that when Wil was only 5 ½ months old, they took him to New York City to see her mother. As soon as they exited the elevator, the normally quiet baby Wil began to scream. There were several other people on that floor, none of whom looked very happy to be there. Once they got her mother away from the floor and outside, Wil calmed down. His screams returned when they took her mother back to her room on that same floor. Taking all of that in, I have always felt that the forgotten souls in retirement homes and hospital rooms, where visitors can be sparse, reflect such intense sadness that surely a baby would feel it. Babies and small children have a sixth sense when it comes to souls, and the son of Sidra was no different. So it stands to reason that she has worked tirelessly volunteering at hospitals, visiting people who have cancer, or who need transplants. She did it in New York, and went straight to Cedars when she arrived in Los Angeles. She was working there when Ava got her transplant. It always fascinates me when I think of people who later become great friends, and have worked or lived in the same spaces. I wonder if they passed each other in the hospital hallways, feeling a sense of familiarity but not being able to put their fingers on it. Maybe glancing back at one another, as one disappears around a corner . . .

And so it also stands to reason that Sidra and Ava would end up in the same dance class and they would meet. And it was there that Sidra saw a void — a sadness — and she stepped right in.

Without question.

Sidra Franklin LoCurto

Artist — Jack of all Trades

Soul Sister

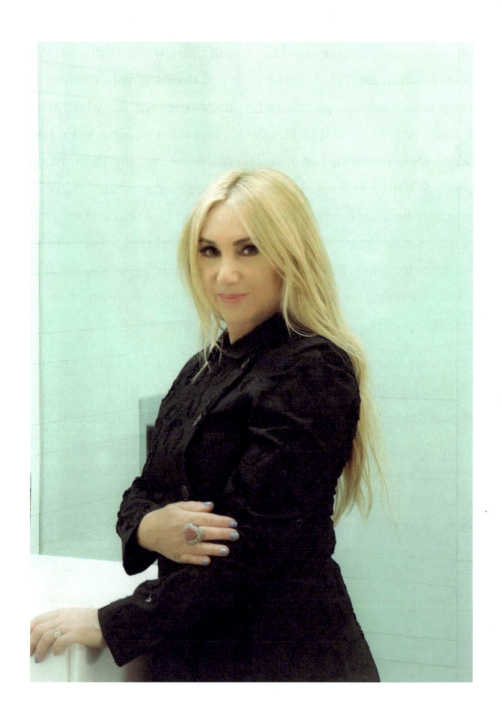

CHAPTER TWENTY-SEVEN
CLARE CULHANE - THERE'S NOTHING MORE BEAUTIFUL THAN A RED-HEADED DANCER

It took me some time to convince Clare to meet me on a video chat. She doesn't like how she looks on her computer. I'm thinking, "Who does?" It's one of those things we have all had to get used to and get over since Covid took over the world. And yet, when the curtain opened, there was the beautiful Clare, just like I remembered her. She has sparkling eyes, now covered by glasses, and a perfect little nose that I swear I saw twitch (ala Samantha Stevens from Bewitched) from time to time while we chatted. Her once red hair is streaked with silver. It's still curly, with just enough bounce, that when she talks about her days performing all over the world, I can see the stage, and the dancer, just as perfectly as if I'd been there back in the '70s. Clare toured with Shirley MacLaine for 7 years, and it was just before that time that she met Ava. And that is where we started our conversation.

"How did you and Ava meet?"

Clare burst into tears. "She's a miracle! I love her so much — you don't understand —" They met in David's 78th Street studio apartment. Clare and David had been together for a long time. Clare walked in and saw Ava baking cookies, wearing her leotard.

She wondered, "Who bakes cookies in a leotard??" Well, Ava does. It was 1974 in New York City and they were a trio of dancers and the best of friends. Ava and David toured with Gloria Gaynor and Clare toured elsewhere, but they always came together when they got back to the city. Clare had an apartment on 85th Street on the West Side, where she always returned, after living in Los Angeles, Las Vegas, after meeting Queen Elizabeth, and finally back to New York. Even as I write this, I think of that Cole Porter song, *Take Me Back to Manhattan*, from the musical, *Anything Goes*. That was Clare then, and it's Clare now. She is living in Florida, biding her time until she can return to her beloved New York, where she met a leotard-wearing, cookie-baking, crazy, fun, miracle of a friend, Ava.

Clare grew up in Huntington, Long Island, a little piece of paradise with waterfront property and some classic New York State Americana buildings and roadways. It has streets that look frozen in time in the 1950s. There are bridges through woods that look like the Headless Horseman's bridge from *The Legend of Sleepy Hollow*. It has harbors, gently speckled with boats, ready for a day trip up or down the coast. Buildings step out of an even further past reimagined with modern awnings and shiny new business names, replacing businesses long ago shut down. Clare spent her summers in Montauk, where the landscape of Huntington gave way to long stretches of beach and craggy rocks with a lighthouse, on which a young girl could dream of a different life for herself, far away from Huntington. And then, as if God heard her thoughts, when she was fifteen, Clare and her mother moved into the city, leaving behind a difficult childhood that culminated in her parents' divorce. They moved into an apartment on East 79th Street and, when she was 16, Clare's mother let her drop out of school so she could dance full time.

Three years after they moved to New York City, Clare's mother died from breast cancer. She was on her own. I cannot imagine the pain of losing my mother, but I feel like her mother must have known. I don't think it was an accident that she moved them to NYC where Clare could flourish as a dancer. She did what she thought was best for her daughter. While many people might not understand the idea of allowing your daughter to drop out of High School, perhaps Clare's mother knew that dance provided an escape for a soul that could not find it elsewhere. When I was young, I too would look out across the river where I grew up, watching the ripples dance away down around the bend, wondering where they got to go . . . There is always a reason, and it is simply not for any of us to judge. For Clare, dancing saved her soul, and her mother knew her soul needed to dance. "My mother was a great woman," she told me. "I had the best mother on Earth. She was a sergeant in World War II. Can you imagine that? Ava is as great a woman to me as my mother."

So that was it. Somehow, the petite, cookie-baking-in-a-leotard woman reminded her of her mother. Perhaps, just that Ava's honest, brash, loving, funny personality gave Clare a sense of belonging. And perhaps that she took no shit, like Clare's World War II vet mother. The one who took her daughter to New York

City and allowed her to do what she needed to do, with total acceptance. And she saw it with Ava's heart. In Clare's mind, she feels she is so blessed, to this very day, to have had two such amazing women in her life. "I'm so lucky . . .", she says, and she starts to cry again.

After her mother died, Clare knew she couldn't stand still. She began to audition, and of course, she got multiple jobs. She did a summer tour of *Promises, Promises*, with Betty Buckley and Donald O'Connor. Her eyes lit up when she talked about it. I was thrilled to hear the names of these Broadway stars and imagined what that could have been like. She danced and performed with Gregory Hines, Dean Martin, and even Roger Moore . . . "But do you know who I got to meet — who even talked to me?" She didn't wait for me to guess. "Gregory Peck! And he shook my hand and looked right at me, and he said, 'There's nothing like a beautiful, red-headed dancer!'" The excitement fell away again. Reminiscing about such an exciting past has its traps. And that, I am sure, is why she keeps moving around in her life, staying busy, trying new things. Staying away from life's traps.

Shirley MacLaine's tour ended in 1983, and Clare continued to work for a while. She got certified as a personal trainer and then quit after a few years. "That was just too much," she tells me, laughing, knowing I have been a personal trainer for over thirty years. "I lost my little apartment in 1996, and I hung out in the city for a couple more years, then I moved to Florida."

Next, we turn our attention to Ava's death, coma, heart transplant, and recovery. Clare cannot talk about that first day when Ava went into cardiac arrest and died in the doorway of her house. David called her every day, to give her a minute-to-minute update on Ava's condition. He told her about every second leading up to the transplant. The stories from the waiting room. The surgery and all of the problems, until Ava was able to speak again. They were so close, she couldn't bear it. "We went through breast cancer together, and her hip replacements, and years and years of romances and dramas. We were best friends. Our hearts were connected. We still talk every single day." Everything is said emphatically. She needs me to understand how deeply they care for each other. "I was never really a wild child, but Ava — well, I kept her grounded. I loved her absolutely unconditionally." There was a history that came across the screen, flowing rapidly through her eyes, that encompassed a lifetime of dancing, laughing, crying, talking, travelling, dining, clubs, classes, stages, opening curtains and closing nights, backstage antics, applause . . . Then back in a class, with a barre and a mirror, new combinations, and watching younger dancers pouring in off the busy streets.

"David, no doubt, made everything into a dramatic story, but we all knew Ava was going to be okay. Because she's Ava. She makes cookies in a leotard."

When Ava was ready to leave the hospital, Mona and Uncle Saul arranged for Clare to come live with her in an apartment in

Westwood. But only for six months. After that, they would have to move out and Clare would have to return to Florida.

Jade came back to live with them. Nurses came and went. Jade was almost 12 years old and she was dying to get out and run or ride or do whatever she could. She would ride her scooter up and down the halls of the Westwood apartment building. And she would go exploring. "We lost her once," Clare confessed to me. "We even had to call the police that time. She was visiting with the neighbors upstairs! We didn't even know she *knew* the people upstairs!" Clare shopped for groceries, made meals, cleaned up, and all the while, they chatted. They watched Two-and-a-Half Men and laughed until their sides hurt. They caught each other up on the lives of mutual friends and ranted about Saul, as the deadline approached . . .

"That six months went by fast."

Ava worked hard to get off the walker and move around on her own. And Clare watched and listened with the patience of an angel and waited for her friend to return to the strong, vibrant dancer she knew. And then, their time was up and Clare went back to Florida. She told me about a short story by Truman Capote called A Day's Work. In the story, Truman Capote's housekeeper, Mary Sanchez, said that when she cleaned his house, there should be no one home. They should leave the money for her with a rolled joint. Clare decided to start a cleaning business and adapted the same rules, minus the joint. She was happy to make everything clean and organized and leave without having to deal with the people who made the mess.

Suddenly, I realized I could talk to this woman forever. To hear the life of a beautiful young girl, who grew up with a pain that she will never speak of. She looked out at an ocean, past the lighthouse on her summer vacation, waiting for an escape. Her mother gave her the freedom to walk away from a conventional life and follow a dream that she knew would save her life. I found that so compelling. She found a friend who believed her story without question, who saw nothing in her but beauty and talent, and supported every adventure she ever went on . . . just like Clare's mom. So when it is difficult to understand Clare's unconditional love for her friend, one would only need to look at what she needed in her own life. Imagine this. No matter where Ava goes in her life, and no matter what she does, or who she is with, someone out there thinks she is a miracle. Someone out there thinks she is one of the two greatest women who has ever lived.

The Captivating Clare.

An unconditional friend, and

A Beautiful Red-Headed Dancer

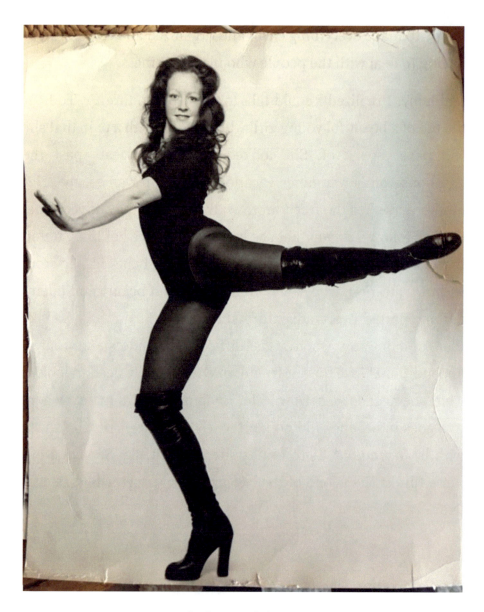

The beautiful Clare

CHAPTER TWENTY-EIGHT
HILARY SUAREZ - THE WARRIOR QUEEN

When she was 9 or 10 years old, Hilary was diagnosed with myocarditis. Myocarditis is the inflammation of the heart muscle, caused by an untreated viral infection. She'd had stomach aches and flu-like symptoms, and bumps in her mouth that travelled down into her throat. She was given antibiotics and told to drink fluids. The infection appeared to have gone away, but in reality, it had travelled down into her body and affected her heart. At USC Medical Center, the first hospital she was transferred to, she stopped breathing. She was then taken to Children's Hospital Los Angeles, where she met her doctors, who would figure everything out.

Hilary sits on our video chat in a red hooded sweatshirt with a headband and her deep brown hair tied up high on her head in a knot. She has the clearest eyes and skin I think I have ever seen. She looks younger than her twenty-one years and probably always will. I am floored by her beauty and her drive to make the world a better place for other people. The beauty streams from her like inner sunshine. It's incredible. She lives in a place of the purest hope.

When she woke up in CHLA, she was confused. She didn't understand why she couldn't be with her family. She was a little girl, suddenly put into a horrible situation, which she would have to live with now. She took a lot of medications, and by the time she was eleven or twelve, her heart had started to settle down. She joined cheerleading and dance. "I got to experience what it was like to be a normal teenager . . ." But then, by the time she was 13, depression began to set in. "I tried to stay positive because I felt normal. I didn't feel sick." But the depression was always there, looming at the edge of her aura. In tenth grade, Hilary was in a mini-mart. "I was alone there when I collapsed. My heart stopped." There are angels everywhere, and I'm sure they were there that day, because someone called for an ambulance and she got back to CHLA. She had a defibrillator implanted, and that became the turning point in her childhood. She became anxious and depressed, feeling sicker every day. "I could feel my body giving up," she told me. "I tried to stay positive, but I couldn't even go to school. I tried, but my chest hurt and I was always short of breath. Therapy helped, but I still just felt like giving up." Once the positivity began to slip away, she felt like she was going to die soon, and she found a way to be okay with that. Her life became a struggle between her own emotions, where she felt that if God made the decision to take her, she was okay — and yet . . .

She wanted to fight.

I am listening to this lovely young woman in her red hoodie, and I cannot imagine her being anything but positive. Looking at her is like looking at Hope in its very soul. There is not an ounce of trepidation in her now, in those extraordinarily clear brown eyes. And then I learn why they are so clear.

Eventually, Hilary entered the hospital as an inpatient. She didn't want to live there, but she wanted a heart. She was there for three months, living in a unit, not allowed to step outside of it. She had tubes in her neck and arms. And the teenager who should have been wearing the latest fashion, crop tops, short shorts, t-shirts, jeans or her cheerleading outfit, was stuck in a hospital gown. Every. Single. Day. Graduation was fast approaching, but there wasn't going to be a prom or a grad night or any of those special times with her classmates. "Sometimes, I would get multiple arrhythmias in a single day. The doctors would try to bump me closer to the top of the transplant list, so I asked them if I should prepare myself to die . . . My parents gave me so much love, and the more love I got from them, the harder I fought." She fought the depression and the fatigue, and she prayed for a heart.

Before I had a chance to ask the tough question — the one about praying for someone else's heart, Hilary offered a response. "I had to ask myself, am I praying for someone else to die so I can get this heart?" But she wasn't. She was only praying that she could have a chance at life. A healthier, stronger life than she had ever had before. She didn't even know what it meant anymore. It had been so long since she had felt normal. On August 7, 2018, at 4:00 am, she woke up. There was no alarm — nothing loud. After she had opened her eyes, a nurse entered the room to tell her she had a phone call. It was her transplant coordinator. And then she heard the words:

"We have a heart for you."

She called her parents, who were already on their way. "I was SO happy!" She still smiles at the memory of it. At 11:00 pm that night, Hilary was being wheeled into surgery. "Everyone hugged me as I rolled down the hallway. I didn't want to let go of their hands. What if . . ."

"I was going to get a brand new life."

The hands fell aside, but I am sure she could feel the love and the warmth and hope that followed her into the operating room. At midnight, they opened her up, and Hilary got her new heart on August 8, 2018. "I woke up after the surgery, and there were IVs everywhere. But I felt no pain. I felt good. I was not scared, and I was healthy. I could *feel* it." Two days after her surgery, Hilary had her stomach tube removed, and she was able to walk, and after a week, there were no tubes or wires. Just the central line. "I felt free!" There she was, not yet 19 years old, and she was telling herself that if she could take baby steps every day, she would get out of the hospital. She left the hospital two weeks later and said this: "It was a new life for me. I felt like nothing could stop me. I took my meds, always, because I was going to make sure that I took very good care of this gift. I am healthy now and grateful every day for my donor and the heart I have been given. I sometimes wonder, was she someone like me? Because of my donor, I am alive. I sent them (the donor family) a letter, but I have not heard back. I must always honor them by taking care of this heart."

Her high school graduation was on FaceTime at the hospital, and now, she is just like every other young lady her age. She likes to hang out with her friends, Andrea, Evanna and Hannah. She said that while most people didn't know what she was going through, these girls were always there for her. When she was first diagnosed, people largely stayed away from her, perhaps not knowing what to say. Her family gave her hope. Her sisters, Monica and Leilani, came to see her in the hospital. Monica's three little kids, Annabelle, Amanda and Adrian, liked to come along. Her family always told her, "You are a warrior. You have so much power!"

That is such a fascinating way to look at Hilary. And I have to say, I agree with them.

So many people have touched Ava's life, but it seems fitting that when I asked Hilary how she knew Ava, she told me that she was doing a fundraiser for her senior project, and at CHLA, she was told about Ava's Heart. Ava came and met her family and friends and gave them goody bags as giveaways for her to pass out for her senior presentation. She raised $500 for Ava's Heart.

She just kept giving, teaching, loving and praying.

I am amazed by this young woman. She wanted to be a marine biologist when she was younger, but through her illness, she found new, clearer call. "Depression changed who I was as a child. My family told me to pray, and therapy helped. The doctors and nurses were incredible. I read about kids who had been through more than what I had, and I came to realize that if they could do it, I could do it. And I had to have faith in my parents." So Hilary is studying to become a registered nurse, and she wants to go into pediatrics.

Clarity. It's all in the eyes.

Some angels are born and some are made. I don't know which Hilary Suarez is, but I know that the day she walks into a child's room who is suffering, she will tell them what she said she would tell her ten-year-old self: "Don't give up. Have faith. Keep Smiling. Fight for what you want."

And they will know that she speaks from the heart.

Hilary Suarez

The Clear-Eyed Warrior Queen and Angel-in-Waiting

Lives in Los Angeles (The City of Angels) with her Family

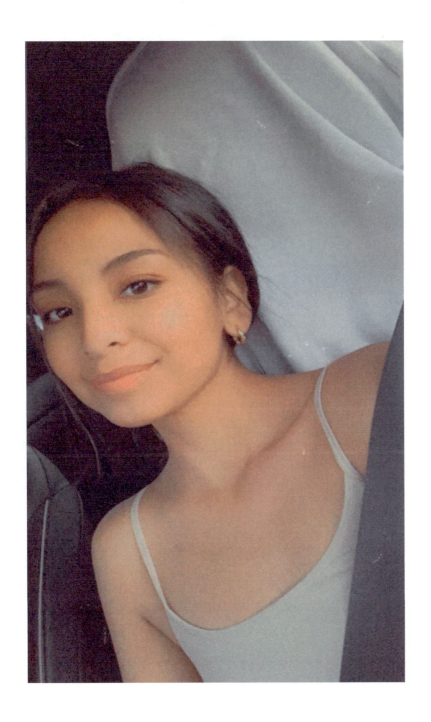

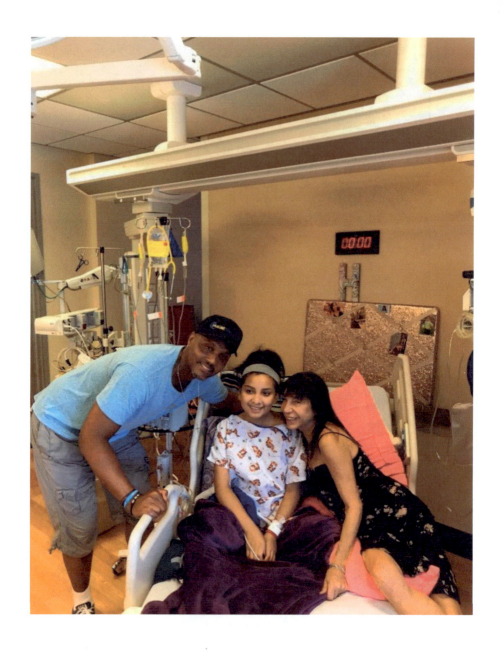

Seejai, Hilary and Ava

CHAPTER TWENTY-NINE
DESIREE HUITRADO & ANDREW JOHN "WISKY SPARROW" SHARP - WILD CHILD IN THE MIDDLE

Desiree is a mom — sometimes she was a single mom, and sometimes she wasn't. She is the kind of person who speaks from her heart, and when the pain comes, she immediately talks about her faith until her voice stabilizes. As I ask her about her personal life, she speaks to me with unabashed honesty. I asked her about her sons, and she tells me a story of when she had her eldest son, Timothy. She and her then husband had needed to go through fertility treatments to try to have another child. When she came home from the doctor to tell her husband she was pregnant, she found him in bed . . . . well . . . not with her, obviously. Pregnant and with a toddler, she turned and walked out the door — and never looked back. The baby she was pregnant with was Andrew. She straightens up a bit when she tells me that story, still standing firmly by her decision. Desiree moves through her life with such grace and with the deepest sense of faith, and in a way that, if you didn't take the time to speak to her, you might miss it. Her youngest son, Michael, is 26. She was a caregiver until she developed a debilitating condition known as Charcot Foot and could no longer work.

I can see the weariness around her face and in her eyes. I entered this interview with very little knowledge of her life or Andrew's. Her voice fails a little as we talk, and she cries from time to time, but she talks about the Lord and her unwavering faith — repeating His words and His will until the tears stop. She struggles, she speaks about faith, she recovers, and we move on. I have always had a good understanding of how faith works, but Desiree is the embodiment of her belief.

Andrew was employed as a sheet metal worker. "He loved working with his hands," she tells me. "He would tinker with anything. Cars. Computers. Clocks. It didn't matter. Before that, when he was little, he played pop-warner football, but his head was too round for the helmet." I laughed at that. I have two daughters with big heads. I get it! For Andrew, it earned him one of his first nicknames — Pumpkinhead. She said he was a happy baby and became a bit of a troublemaker. We laughed at the idea that being a mischievous boy could get you in so much trouble. Again, I think of my own son when his elementary school administrators raised their voices to me and insisted I get him "tested," so they could put him in a box and label him. I took him to the doctor. Three times actually. They told me they were formally diagnosing him as a "100% pure boy". Desiree smiled at that. "Yes", she said. "Andrew was "all boy" too. He was mischievous and kind, and he was friends with everyone. He never held a grudge — always smiling and was such a lovable person . . ."

She starts to cry.

Andrew loved motorcycles. He crashed his first one, and he bought another one. When he crashed that one, he bought another one. This last one was his fourth. It was registered to Desiree, so on October 7, 2020 when a Toyota Forerunner towing a tractor-trailer collided with Andrew, the police knocked on Desiree's door at midnight. Her middle son was airlifted to Riverside Community Hospital. She arrived at the hospital within hours and was met with the list of his injuries, which, for the sake of his two young daughters, Savannah and Jazzy, I will not list here. No mother should have to see her child like that, and no child should have to see a parent like that. Andrew had become a father when he was very young and moved between the two worlds of an adventurous, carefree young man and his desire to be a responsible father. His friends called him "Wisky Sparrow." Desiree didn't know why, but they all had funny nicknames. I looked it up. It's a band in Mississippi — but they are Whiskey Sparrow. It is spelled slightly differently. Then I looked up "sparrow" — and there it was. A sparrow represents the self-expression and freedoms of those who choose to live outside the limits of society. Even with its small structure, it symbolizes strength and power, and it represents the courage and caution that you should express in your life. It embodies friendliness and joy and compassion. Sailors used to tattoo a sparrow on their bodies so that if they died in the middle of the sea, the sparrow would take their soul to Heaven. "He was my wild child," Desiree told me. Her eyes drifted away from the camera for a moment. Wisky Sparrow, as it turns out, suited Andrew perfectly.

Desiree looked upon each of her sons with equal but different adoration. Raising three boys — sometimes alone — could not have been easy. It's written all over her. Andrew loved life and wanted to live it. He would call her from Colorado, or Washington, to let her know he was there. Then he would be back. On his last birthday, he posted a message on his FaceBook page. It read as follows: *Today 30 years ago, my Mom was in the hospital. Still today, she says I am a pain. 30 years came too fast. Love you Mom, Always Your Middle.* She has that post memorized, and she tells me, "*Me!* He wrote that to me on his birthday." She is surprised at his reverence for her. I cannot understand how she says that so humbly, raising these boys who love her so much.

When she left the hospital later that day, they gave her his helmet to take home with her. Inside, she found a picture that he always carried with him. It was a picture of her.

On October 20, 2020 at 3:33 pm, Andrew John "Wisky Sparrow" Sharp was declared brain dead. Desiree tells me, "In June, I sent him a story of a mom who posted her son's mangled motorcycle on the internet. I miss him."

Desiree and Andrew's father donated his organs.

"I miss him," she says again.

She met Ava through One Legacy because she needed help with Andrew's burial. "Ava was so kind — she just got us what we needed. I couldn't think about what was happening. I just followed the path that the Lord had put in front of me. And Ava was on that path."

Desiree hopes that whoever gets his heart is just like him — or becomes just like him — free-spirited, kind, loving and giving, with a hint of a wild child in them. She spends her nights awake, shopping online. She has all of Andrew's Christmas presents, already wrapped, in her closet. She washed and boxed up all of his clothes, sparing a Broncos jersey for his daughter, Jazzy.

Our conversation stops for a moment. Desiree looks around her room, and I can tell she feels like maybe she hasn't said enough. That I can't understand who he was. But I do. At the time of our conversation, Andrew had only been gone for 8 days. I understand that this perfectly imperfect boy, her "Middle", who returned a mother's unconditional love, was gone. But I also know that she knew how much he loved her. He was the kind of person who was not afraid to tell the whole world how he felt. That is a rare gift, especially for such a young man. Andrew's daughters, both exquisitely beautiful, excelled in school beyond his wildest dreams. He was extraordinary, and in the gifts he bestowed on other people, he will continue to live.

"Can I tell you about something else?" She asks me. And then I hear about Desiree's perfect day. It was Thanksgiving 2019. She had all three of her sons home for a holiday, along with her grandchildren. It snowed in Victorville, and for the briefest moment in time, Desiree looked at her whole family surrounding her, and she had perfection.

"It was a perfect day — you know? It was perfect."

Andrew John "Wisky Sparrow" Sharp

The Wild Child Stuck in the Middle,

Flying to Heaven on the Back of a Sparrow

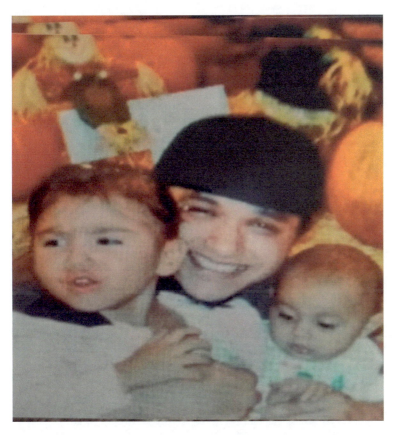

Andrew "Wisky Sparrow" Sharp with his daughters

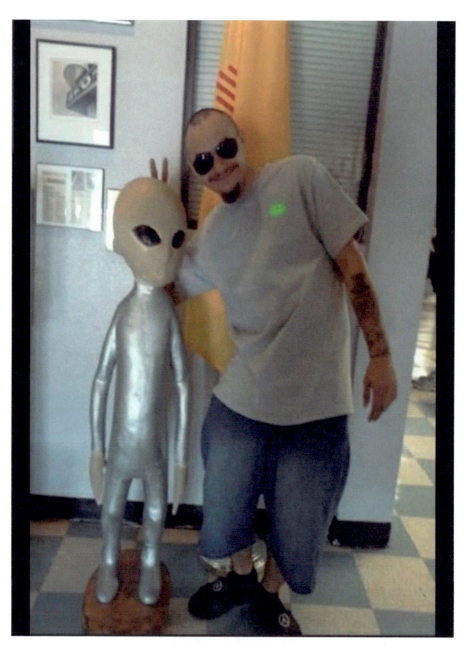

Andrew making peace with an alien

CHAPTER THIRTY
SEAN TIWANAK - KEEPER OF A SURFING HEART, ARMED WITH A UKULELE

There is a saying that "if you feel like you've been for a crazy ride around the mulberry bush, then you have just met an Aries" . . . Or, you've just met Sean Tiwanak. He is the quintessential ball of energy. He is the essence of Hawaii and of positivity. There is never enough time to speak to him because he will always have more to say. But I have learned, through this writing journey, that sometimes when people have a lot to say, it is because the world is not really listening. Such are the words of Sean . . . of Joe Lafferty . . . of Anurag Saksena . . . of Ava. "I contacted Ava prior to coming to Los Angeles," Sean tells me. "We went for a walk the other day. We are kindred spirits. She has given me so much information and comfort. What she accomplishes is beyond even her. She touches so many peoples' lives. She always offers me her house, but as long as I can manage alone, I do."

The first thing Sean shows me in our interview is a picture of Zach, his donor. "There is no me without him," he tells me. "His family told me he was like Superman and that he loved surfing." And boom! There it was. "I felt an immediate miracle. It happened quickly for me, and while I believe firmly in medicine, I also believe in spirituality." I understood by this, that Sean was talking about the spirit world, not just spirituality. He tells me a story about something that happened in their home in Hawaii when he was young. "We were living on the Big Island. I woke up one night and I saw a dark figure go into my brother's room, and he started choking. Then the figure was in my room and I sent it away. The next morning, my Mom asked me about the dark figure - if I had seen it. She had seen it too. In my young-boy mind, I thought that I had protected us, but when my Mom told me she had seen it too, I realized it was my Mom who was protecting us. It wasn't me. It was her." Sean understands a spiritual, almost mystical world. He has smelled Zach in his sleep and has been awakened with full knowledge of Zach's presence. Some people may think that's impossible, but they are not in his situation. Feeling the presence of the very soul of another person within yourself is the measure of transference. Some say it is dangerous, but Sean, says, "I am a living memorial. Zach is gone, but his heart still beats inside of me." He kisses Zach on his forehead and puts the picture back on a mantle, where a single candle burns eternally.

As we move into the story of what happened to him, there are two distinct chapters. Sean is a jack of all trades and a master of music. That is his essence. But there is a medical side to him as well. It's the side that knew something was desperately wrong when a doctor told him he had asthma. And then there is the side that loved a woman named Maile. "Maile is a pua. She's a flower." And things weren't going well with Maile. When she turned away from him, he could feel his heart breaking.

He was working in construction, when he got injured and could no longer work. Never one to be held back, he got a degree as a respiratory therapist, specializing in heart disease and cardiomyopathy. He also got his business degree. His father was a prominent businessman in Hawaii and he felt he had to be the most well-rounded he could be. He married Maile and they moved to Seattle, where he was a respiratory therapist and she worked in legal document discovery. They moved to Philadelphia, then to Reno. He wanted to be an entrepreneur, so he started a contracting business in ceramic tile installation. "One of my employees wanted to be my right-hand guy. One day, he brought ceviche to my office for lunch. But, you know, he didn't look so good. Against my better judgment, I ate the ceviche, and as I ate, he was telling me how his whole family was sick. Maile hated that I was so generous," he says, laughing. "One day later, I had horrible abdominal problems, which then moved into my lungs. When I would get up to walk somewhere in the house, I would be gasping for air. That's when the doctor told me I had asthma, but I knew she was wrong. I had been a respiratory therapist. I had CHEYNE breathing, and that can lead to cardiac arrest. It woke me up over and over. I went to the ER and my lungs sounded like they were crackling. I convinced them to give me a chest x-ray and it showed I had a severely enlarged heart. I knew I was in end-stage viral cardiomyopathy." His body was attacking the disease by killing his heart muscle. Sean got listed for his heart in 2020. "They want to know about your finances. And you can't be sick at all. Nothing." His pulmonary pressures were too high, and it took him 10 days to get stabilized after arriving at Cedars Sinai in Los Angeles. The first heart that came through for him was rejected by the doctors, and then he got Zach's heart — a perfect match.

That was the medical part.

The spiritual journey was another story. "You can have broken heart syndrome," he said. "Maile was my second wife, and technically, we are divorced. We had expectations when we were married. I am Mulder and she is Scully. I am sensitive and she is pragmatic and logical. I felt like my broken heart just waited there for so long, and then it just couldn't wait anymore." He had a mother named Mary, who had cultivated a strong sense of spirituality in him, and Maile could not relate, spiritually speaking. "When I was first sick, I was sinking lower than low. I was in such despair! My parents brought me a piece of a Holy Shroud of the nun who took care of Father Damien, who cared for the lepers on the island of Molokai. Her name was Marianne Cope. I kept the piece of her shroud. She was very strong. I began to play the piano out of desperation to find something. So the emotional healing began while I was still sick. And then, everything fell apart in 2015, and I left Maile for a few months. I felt that everyone abandoned me. I was in a hospital in Reno while my Mom was dying in Hawaii in a hospice center. She was one of the last patients there before they closed their doors forever. My music was playing over the speakers there when she died. I was carrying an unexplainable agony — I was doped up in Reno and my mother was dying of brain cancer in Hawaii."

It all sounded like the journey of someone who was searching for his place in the world. He was hurting and scared and desperate to be heard. He could not be with Mary when she died, but she came to him in his dreams. "I had to explain to her that she was dead. She did not understand — or agree." His life has been a series of signs that he reads through his music. He tells the story of an accident he had had while driving a motorcycle. He was listening to the song, "What a Day for a Daydream," when he fell asleep and crashed the bike. He was pinned to a guardrail, but he missed all of the poles. "There are guardian angels. I know that. There is my Mom, and there is Maile." When he had his transplant, he feared he would never be able to surf again. But Zach's parents told him how much Zach loved to surf. And he knew that everything was going to be okay. He has learned to slow down and take better care of himself and his new heart. "It is difficult to make people understand what this all means. Someone else's heart is beating inside of you because yours broke."

Sean is a man surrounded by angels. Some from the past and some, like Maile, who, while on her own spiritual journey, has found him again.

He offers to sing for me. I, of course, accept. And so he sings that song, the medley of "Somewhere Over the Rainbow/It's a Wonderful World" with his ukulele. And it turns out it's the song that made his good friend, Israel Ka'ano'i Kamakawiwo'ole, or Bruddah Iz, famous. It's so beautiful. And may I just say how

221

honored I was to be listening to a survivor of life and love — a medical miracle, as all organ transplant recipients are, singing on my screen with his ukelele, as I am sure his mother Mary and his friend Bruddah Iz looked on. There is a lot to say about Sean. A story that flows from Mauna Kea, through the sea to the Mainland and back again. He has been saved by a wave, by his mother and by Maile — and by his music. "Zach's birthday is June 13," he tells me. "We want to go surfing. I know that I am blessed, and when you are blessed, you also carry a burden. You have to have that to keep you humble. We are going to paddle for ten to fifteen minutes until we get out there, one arm's length at a time. That's how things are now. One arm length at a time."

I imagine there will be a sound of lapping water as he swims out there. The clear blue-green of the ocean below a sky dappled with fluffy white clouds, and the green mountain sides of the island behind him. The air will be still, except for the occasional sea bird, and, as he paddles on his board, one arm's length at a time, Zach's heart will beat with the anticipation of the first of many waves they will catch together.

Sean Tiwanak

Master of Music

Keeper of Zach's Heart

As He Tries to Re-Capture Maile's Heart

Singer — Songwriter — Soul Surfer

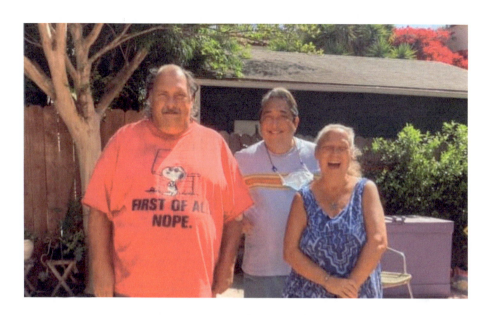

Jerry, Sean and Robin get to meet

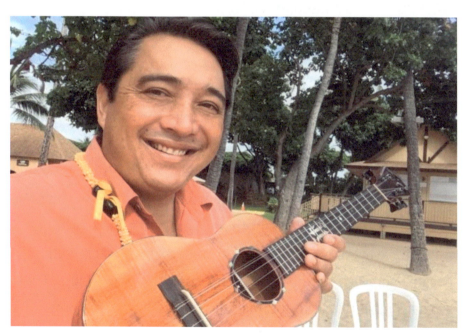

Sean with his Ukulele

CHAPTER THIRTY-ONE
ZACHARY NEWSOME AND ROBIN & JERRY KOCH - A HEART THAT BEATS IN A BLUE BIRD, ON A RAY OF SUNSHINE, AND ON A PERFECT WAVE . . . STILL

It's a difficult thing to try to piece together someone's life and write about it in a few pages, just trying to get people to understand who they are or were — why they are important and what their contribution to Ava's story is. Each one of their stories is worthy of a novel, at the very least, and Zach was no exception. The first thing his step-father, Jerry said to me was, "That's the important thing. Get people to be donors. However they can be". And that is the important thing. It has resonated throughout these chapters: Without the donor, there is no recipient. No lives are saved where one is lost. But with each donor's story, comes the life of a vibrant young man or woman, who was strong and healthy and who loved life in their own way. A life that all of us might have had. The story is told in contrast to the recipients, who became very sick or who lived their entire lives with illness. These are lives most of us cannot imagine. But Zach was different.

Zach was born on June 13, 1994 and he was only 26 years old when a life-ending seizure interrupted his plans. And he had some wonderful plans. He wanted to be an entrepreneur. He made custom-designed leather wallets. He was a talented gardener, and he studied finances and corporate law. "He planted an apple tree right outside," Robin tells me. "And he planted it from a single apple seed from an apple he had eaten. You can see it out there," Jerry chimes in. "It's getting really big!" They called him Superman, because they saw him as a young man of extraordinary strength and resolve. The room behind them is filled with Zach's belongings, like he will be stepping back through the door any minute. I see the poster in the corner with his picture in the middle of it. Up in the sky, with fluffy white clouds and rays of light from Heaven streaming through them — like he is an angel.

Zach and his sister, Tiffany were fourteen years apart. Tiffany had been living with their biological father, Leroy when Zach was born. When Zach was 18 months old, Tiffany had suggested that it would be best for him to live with Leroy as well, so he was sent to live in South Carolina. Zach bounced around between the homes of his father, his grandfather (Robin's father) and later, Tiffany and her husband. The disciplinary issues that arose were not that surprising. When Leroy passed away in 2001, Zach returned to Southern California. There had been allegations of abuse on the part of Robin's father, and Zach needed a place to heal. After years of instability, he was now a mischievous 9-year-old, who had no love for school or discipline. He was a little boy, returning to parents he was not used to. Jerry and Robin did their very best to cultivate a healthier diet and a supportive homelife for Zach. They rolled with the temper tantrums and the mood swings, until Zach was finally able to start vocalizing what his issues were. He had trouble breathing, and a doctor told him it was asthma. He had excessive knee pain, and the doctor told him it was Osgood-Schlatter disease, and later they told him it was Hoffa Fat in his knees. Regardless, he lived with a fair amount of pain, not really knowing why or having any definitive answers as to what was happening to him. He started to play baseball and volleyball, rode skateboards and loved to fish. He was becoming a regular Southern California kid. But none of that was to last. A pain that started in his left leg began to slowly but surely move throughout his body, and was later determined to be Complex Regional Pain Syndrome, which is characterized by a pain that is noticeably more severe than the injury that had initially caused it. It can stem from anything like a sprained ankle to a heart attack or stroke. In Zach's case, his seizures started *after* the diagnosis. He lived a large part of his life managing pain and trying to deal with whatever happened to him as a young child. It is often said that people create mechanisms to deal with trauma, even if those mechanisms are based on other body pain. That is not to say that Zach's issues weren't real — quite the opposite. He had to place his trauma somewhere, and while there may be thousands of doctors who do not agree with this assessment, I think his parents *would* agree. The pain has to go *somewhere*.

As Jerry tells me the saga of Zach's seizures, from first to last — 8 in all — I notice that Robin's eyes have drifted away from their computer screen. She is looking somewhere off to her left, but I can see her eyes are filled with tears. My heart drops, because I have spoken to numerous family members of donors by this point, and I know that look. I wish I could reach through the computer and wrap my arms around her, but all I can do is ask her if she is okay and if she would like to continue. "Yes," she says. "Sometimes I just have to cry." For Jerry, he never thought of himself as Zach's stepfather — nor did Zach. They were father and son, and that is evident in Jerry's pain. "I never really even thought of being a stepfather. I just asked him to call me Dad and he did. That's just who we were."

Robin sounds like she has an accent, but it's actually a speech impediment, because of a learning issue. But to me, she is incredibly clear. She is a mother who loved her children and lost them for some years, through circumstances beyond her control. She was deeply affected by Zach's pain and by the fact that she could not help him or give him answers as to where it was coming from. She trusted the medical community to care enough to figure out what was going on with him, but he ended up dying. The one thing I am sure of, is that people who are different from most of us on one level, are far more advanced than us on other levels. After Zach passed away, she could feel him wrapping his arms around her, hugging her, while she did the dishes at her kitchen sink. She feels him and smells him. She senses him outside by the apple tree he planted in their yard, and she knows he is everywhere around her. She tells me that her own mother used to feed the bluebirds up north where she lived. "We don't have any bluebirds here, but a couple of weeks after Zach died, there was one right here in our yard, flying around the apple tree. I know it was my mother letting me know she was with him now. Just a couple of weeks before he died," she tells me, "we had this goldfish. It had lived for 7 years. It died, and Zach went and cleaned the tank and got it all ready for a new fish. But I just couldn't get new ones. But now we've got two. He worked so hard to get everything ready for me to have new fish, so we decided to do it. And they are beautiful! I love them, because I feel like he is here, too." I looked at their Facebook post about the fish tank, and the thing that struck me was the Little Mermaid sitting down in one corner of the tank, because like Ariel, Robin is someone who believes that things are going to get better. She feels her son in every piece of her life — in every corner of their home and yard. I honestly don't know if I would have such strength.

His seizures started on Father's Day in 2018. "I was there to catch him for all of them except the last one," Jerry says. "That day, I went to watch television with my mother, and when I came back, he had collapsed on the floor. My mother did CPR and we did everything we could to try to bring him back. But the seizure was too strong. They told us there was no brain activity, and they spoke to us about donating his organs. I have to say I really credit the doctor for explaining it all to us and we knew Zach would want to help people. He was always helping people. He donated his heart, his kidneys and his liver. He saved four lives." Robin smiles as she shows me the necklace One Legacy sent to her. They are so proud of their son. And it is with exceptional bravery that they continue his legacy by promoting the importance of organ donation. "At Norco High School, we share his story, and people are beginning to recognize the donation process. A friend recently passed from cancer, and although they could not use those organs because of cancer, they could donate the corneas — so they did. And they told us it was because of our story and our bravery."

Jerry pauses. "We don't feel brave."

But they are.

Zach had a 1974 Volkswagen Bug, which he called "The Journey". It's a strangely fitting name for a young man who collected pins from everywhere he visited with Jodi, his girlfriend of nine years. He continues his journey through the lives of each of the four people he saved. Jodi could not go to his memorial, again, for reasons that are not mine to share. But I imagine the pain she must have felt at his loss was equal to that of his family. She has pins and memories and photos, but they are a far cry from being wrapped in the arms of the man she loved. As for The Journey, Jerry cruised it down to the beach for the memorial. Ava's Heart had paid for Zach's cremation. Zach's ashes were inside and Jerry gave everyone a small portion of them. There is a photograph from the memorial of Robin is standing out in the water, her fingers outstretched, as Zach's ashes left her open hands and floated away in the waves. She faces out to the endless expanse. Maybe she is asking a mermaid to take care of him. In the final photo, there are those God clouds again, darkened by the impending night. Shafts of light from a setting sun burst through them and onto the water, where a couple of surfers sit on their boards, waiting for one last wave before darkness falls. I am sure that there was single ash that clung to the board of one of those surfers, hoping to catch that one last wave too.

"Without Ava," Jerry tells me, "I don't know what we would have done." She doesn't always get to meet the donor and the recipient, but this time, she did.

Zach's Journey will continue in the experiences of his recipients, three of whom had reached out to Jerry and Robin, including Sean Tiwanak. Zach was Sean's heart donor. When I wrote Sean's chapter, there was an intermixing of his story and Zach's. He truly feels Zach in his soul, like Robin feels Zach all around her. "Sean is closing this chapter in his life," Jerry tells me. Although they are sad, they are very clear about Sean continuing on his own journey and living his own life. "He wants to get back to Hawaii and to Maile. But we are going to meet him this week. We are going to hear Zach's heart beating."

And *that* is the magic of the donor. Life goes on — for one more song — for one more wave — for one more ray of sunshine — and for one more hug at the kitchen sink.

One Love.

Zach Newsome

Entrepreneur, Gardener, Surfer

Reviving The Journey

With the Wind that Blows Through the Apple Tree in The Backyard

His Giving Heart Still Beats

Donor

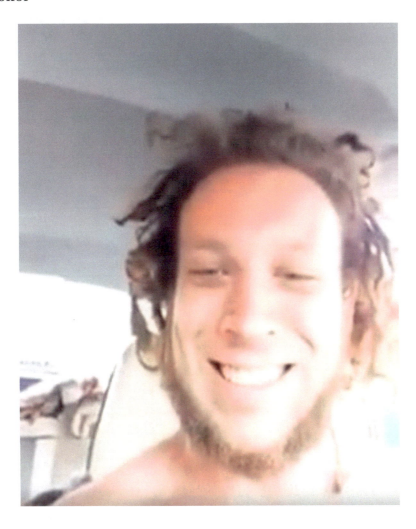

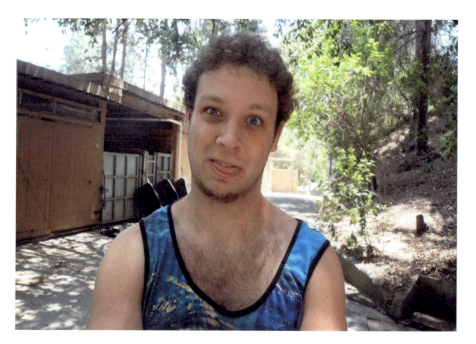

Zach is being silly!

In Hawaiian Mythology, there is a belief that after death, the body would transform into a shark, and it would protect and steer fish towards their family.

CHAPTER THIRTY-TWO
AT THE END OF THE DAY

Ava:

I am left with a feeling of serenity in my life — not because I have come to any end or to any perfectly suitable conclusions that I could bestow on anyone, but because when I get those multiple daily calls, I realize what a giant leap I have taken. There is a voice on the phone, asking me to help them. They are frightened by what is to come, or they have lost someone close to them, and they just need to bury their loved one with dignity. To those who are frightened, I acknowledge that I didn't have the "before". I was already in a coma and the decision was made for me by my doctors and their staff. But I tell them my story, because it is relevant and because it provides hope for a life afterward. I cannot make any promises to those people about their own lives, but I can promise a place for them to call home so that they can at least get there. And at a time where promises are scarce, it gives a sense of comfort to each of them and a sense of fulfilling a promise I made to God a long time ago.

To the voice on the other end of the line who has lost a loved one after that person has saved other lives with the gift of their organs, I tell them I am so sorry for their loss and I can say with equal measure, "Thank you for the gift." I cannot relieve their sadness, but I can take a burden off of their shoulders by helping with the final expenses of their loved ones.

There is a measure of calm in my life because while I have so much more to do, I know that this is being accomplished through my own promise to God. I was not a person who came into this as a wealthy philanthropist. I came at it with nothing but my own shark heart and a desire to right a wrong in the world.

At the end of the day, I have the people I love around me. My family has shifted slightly, as I continue onto my Life's path with my beautiful Jade. She is strong and sassy, always present, and always beautiful to me, inside and out. She is grown and moving to New York City to achieve her own dreams — flying high, as I always dreamed she would. I thank God for allowing me to see that. Across the table from me, I have my friends with whom I am writing this book. They work meticulously, tirelessly . . . until another call comes in. I break from our circle to talk to someone new. I have seen her request on my website and set up cremation services for her daughter, who was a donor. Another life was lost and four lives were saved.

Life doesn't always work out like we think it should and definitely not as we would have wanted it to. I would not have chosen a heart transplant, but I am so grateful for where I am now. I have met so many people that I would not have otherwise met, had this not happened to me first. This book is but a snapshot of some of the lives I am honored to have had become a part of my own. Our paths crossed through a common miracle. And now, every once in a while, when my phone rings, it is someone I was able to help, just checking in.

"I was thinking about you the other day, Ava. How have you been?" . . .

Nothing is perfect . . . My life isn't.

Life can turn on a dime . . . mine did.

But here is what I know. There is something else on the horizon — always. It may not be easy and the path may seem long, or even impossible at times. Whatever happens, more possibilities always arise and hope always present because hope is a choice.

I will continue to love in my life, though it may not be perfect. I will continue to be a mother, for as long as God allows me to, and then I will watch her from the sky.

My love, my Jade, the doctors and nurses and everyone who works in the transplant community, and my eternal friends, my donor . . . everyone I have met on my journey . . . have brought me back to Life.

Donate. Everywhere you can. Anytime you can. However you can.

Donate.

And with that, I fly through the air, on wings that I borrowed from an angel. I plunge into a deep blue sea — so blue that it cannot be replicated — and I swim . . . fast and free. My heart beats with a rhythm that is strong and even and calm. My heart beats . . .

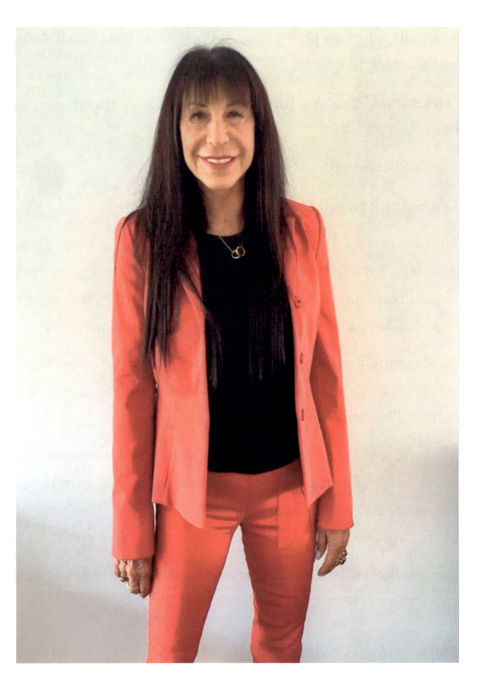

Ava today

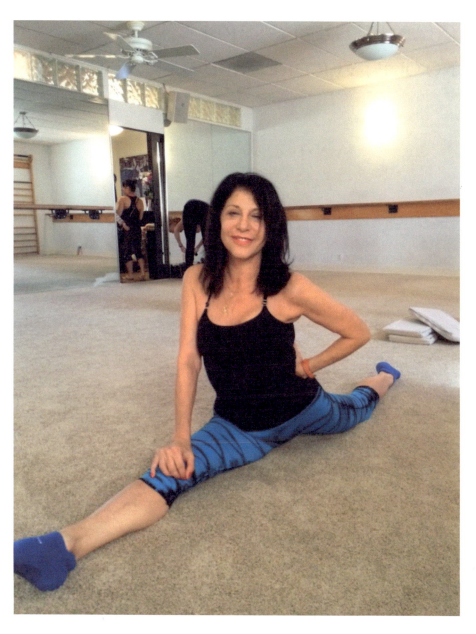

Post-transplant, getting back in shape

CHAPTER THIRTY-THREE
NO ONE EVER DREAMED

No One Ever Dreamed

I never dreamed

As I danced through the orchard

At night, in a pale nightgown

That my heart would break

As I waltzed through life . . .

As I waltzed, and the moon went down

No One ever dreams

Of a second chance

Before the first is ever taken

But as I danced through the orchard

I dreamed of you

A glimpse, a flutter — I was shaken

My second chance at Love — at Life

Came in a flash —

Unexpected

You were there

When I died, then I lived

A love that made me feel protected

No one ever dreams

Of love found, then lost

With the words, "I want you to find another",

So I danced through the orchard

In search of your love

But I was alone, without any lover

Don't ask me to find

Someone to love me

It's you of whom I have dreamed

I never imagined

As I danced late that night

Of a life so far from what it then seemed

Your arms wrapped around me

Our bodies entwined

Forever — Is what I desired

For no one ever dreamed

Of dancing alone

In the orchard, where I was inspired.

I turned and I jumped

As the music played,

Filling the night

Because no one ever dreamed

Of what was coming next

So we danced into the morning light.

CHAPTER THIRTY-FOUR
JADE - LITTLE GIRL LOST, FOUND — SHE PIROUETTES ALL AROUND

My little girl is eleven, and that is how old Jade was when Ava died. It was all such a shock, I am hard-pressed to remember when exactly I first saw Jade after that day — but I know it was in the hospital. I had spent several nights sleeping there, going to work, training clients, showering at the gym, and returning to my vigil at the hospital. I had two of my own children at that time. Jazz, who was a couple of years younger than Jade, and Dakota, who was four years younger. But I had to be there. I was sitting with Mona, when I heard that familiar voice, rambunctious and entertaining. I looked up. Jade's messy, sandy blonde hair was in a ponytail and her little golden freckles practically sparkled. She was wearing her riding clothes, and she began practicing pirouettes on the hallway floors. I remember wondering how much she had been told — maybe nothing — I didn't know — but as I watched her twirl, I thought Ava was inside of her right now, dancing down the hushed hallways of the Saperstein Building. But it wasn't Ava. It was Jade, doing anything she could do to avoid the truth of what was happening. She must have been so scared. And then I noticed that not one single person was comforting her and I realized that the continuous swirling made it impossible for her to focus on where she was. And on why she was there. She was probably just thinking, *"Don't fall!"*

To get a glimpse of who Jade truly was and is, Ava and I sat and talked just about Jade for several hours. Jade did not want to talk about what had happened. Twelve years later, it is still too painful for her. I am not a psychologist, and I don't profess to be one. I am a mom and I cannot imagine my little girl going through what Jade did. My little girl's name is Indie. She was born almost exactly one year after Ava's heart transplant. At almost nine and eleven years younger than her siblings, she spends her days running errands with me and reading me the things she writes in school. She can get bored and cranky sometimes, and other times she wants to snuggle until she falls asleep. She has nightmares and comes into our bedroom and climbs into our bed. She plays sports and likes to bake cookies. She chats with her friends and they all sit up giggling into the wee hours of the morning on their phones. Jade was in that world of friends and experiences and sports and music. Just like my little Indie and me. It was Jade and Ava against the world. I cannot imagine leaving her alone in the world.

Ava told me, "You know, when Jade was five years old, she asked me, 'Do you think the reason God doesn't want to come down to Earth is that he is afraid to see what he created?' What makes a five-year-old think like that?" Jade is a thoughtful human being. I think it was what made her such an extraordinary equestrian. She completely understood animals, on a deeper level than most humans would even bother to comprehend. I went to see Jade ride one afternoon. To this very day, I have never seen anyone become one with an animal like Jade was with Ranja. I recently saw a picture of her mid-jump, and it brought tears to my eyes. I used to watch Jade climb through the windows of Ava's car like it was a series of caves she was exploring. She was always either coming or going from the barn. Ava's car was strewn with Jade's stuff, and I noticed a small, brown horse sitting on the dashboard. I asked about the horse. It looked like it was glued there and seemed to be, therefore, hazardous to the driver's line of sight. Ava said, "Oh, you know the singer Beck? Well, his brother's wife gave that to Jade." Ava was lifelong friends with Beck's stepmother. The strange part is that I am from Winnipeg, and so is Beck's sister-in-law. She was one of my best friends growing up. "Are you talking about Lisa Mark?" Jade swung back from the roof of the car through the window and into her seat. "How do you know Lisa Mark?"

It's a small world.

The point of it all was that Jade was the kind of kid that everyone knew. Even another girl from Wildwood Park in Winnipeg. She was funny and pretty and boisterous and so incredibly talented. And on that horse . . . well, that was sheer perfection.

That's where she was meant to be when her life was interrupted. She was meant to sing and dance until the music came to an abrupt halt.

Before Ava went into the hospital, when her body was blowing up and she didn't know what was happening to her, she had asked a woman who she didn't know very well if Jade could stay with her, in case anything happened to her. That woman was Linda York, who to this very day, is one of the calmest, kindest people I have ever met. She lived in a tiny cottage in Santa Monica. It was safe and warm and Jade and her little dog Pebbles stayed there with Linda. So Linda was my next phone call.

Linda did not have a past with Ava. They were new friends. Linda's days revolved around Jade. She made sure she saw the people who were important to her, so that she could just be Jade. They would walk down to the beach in the mornings before school and spend time together. She would do some riding, and sometimes Linda's granddaughter, Beatrice, would be with them. Jade was very gentle with Beatrice, who was only 2 or 3 years old at the time. Linda made sure that she was surrounded by love and a little family and exceptional kindness and caring. Linda had a pink silk shirt with green polka dots, which Jade slept in. She would lie on her tummy and Linda would rub her back until she fell asleep. Linda worked on ways to keep her anchored. They would come up with ways for her to stay in touch with Ava. For Jade, her emotions went on pause. There was no future and no past. She just existed in her own world with Linda and Beatrice and Pebbles, in a little cottage by the sea. She asked Linda once, "Did you ever have something that hurt so much; you couldn't talk?" Yes, Linda did. She had come to an understanding, through her own life, loves and losses, that relationships don't end just because someone is not there anymore. They go on. But to Jade, everything just seemed like it had stopped. She told Ava some years later that she remembered thinking that she was either going to die, or she needed walls up to protect herself. She had to close herself in. So that was what she did. She didn't want to be put off by people who didn't want her, and she didn't want to be with Michael. She didn't trust him. She was never cruel about it — but she was Ava's child. Not Michael's. And, even as an eleven-year-old, she knew that he had his own demons to deal with. Late at night, she would call Ava's cell phone and leave her messages, sometimes asking where she was, and sometimes to say good-night and tell her that she loved her. When Ava finally woke up from her coma and got her phone back, she listened to every single one.

What was also clear to Jade is that she had lost her lifestyle. Not that she was a materialistic child, but her stability was gone. Her life with a formidable mother who could make anything happen, had evaporated. Everything seemed uncertain. All of the things that she had been groomed for were gone. She was an equestrian without a horse, and a gifted actress and singer who had lost her confidence. The barn and school faded away with equal distance. The school was simply not high on her list of priorities. Survival was . . . and she fell behind. Jade was a brilliant girl, with a mind that saw people exactly for who they were, without an ounce of judgment. But she knew who wanted to be around her and who didn't. She knew who was safe, and who wasn't. Those weren't qualities she learned about in any classroom. As the reality of a new life began to emerge, more and more of her options were shut down. So she could rely only on herself. And she understood what she needed to sacrifice to keep Ava alive. That was the mind of eleven-year-old Jade. And she stayed that way. She got stuck.

Linda was a respite for Jade. Jade used to call her "Leonard". I had forgotten that. It cracked me up every time Jade spoke to or about Linda — or Leonard. At just eleven years old, Jade lived in constant fear that if anything else happened to Ava, she would not know how to take care of it. She did not think about the future other than asking Linda if she would always be able to come back to live with her, no matter what happened with Ava.

Once Ava was released from the hospital, Jade just wanted to be near her. To help her and take care of her. And also, perhaps, to try to take up where she left off in her childhood. But, despite everything she went through, and all of the places they moved after selling the house, Jade never once complained about where she was, as long as she was with her mom.

Ava recently spoke to the kids of a man who was staying at Ava's House, getting ready for their father's transplant. These kids were older than Jade was when Ava had her transplant, but it was clear that they were stunned — still stuck at the moment when their father had gotten so sick. And they had their mother and they had each other. There is the healing of the patient, but also the healing of the families. There is a moment for these families when they step out into the world with the possibility that their loved ones will no longer be there to walk through life with them.

Jade took that step alone. When she was eleven.

Jade was, and still is, a young woman who has so much love and admiration for her mother but who is still in protection mode for her. She never accepted a gift, if she felt that it would make Ava feel bad for not being able to provide it. She was deathly afraid that Ava wouldn't be coming back, so she allowed her life to become one of deferred dreams and sacrifices.

Jade is twenty-four years old now. She is a stunning beauty, with long, dark hair and big, green eyes. She has moved to New York City to follow her dreams. Somewhere along the way, she found the strength to heal; her own healing has been peripheral to Ava's for so many years. Jade never lost faith in her mother. Now she is ready to reach out for her own life.

But there will always be a thread that connects these two women. As far away as Jade may roam, I will always remember her rushing out of the room where we wrote this book, flipping her thick, dark mane of hair as she flashes a smile. "Mom!" She calls out. She is slightly impatient. "Where are the car keys?"

As it should be . . .

The messy-haired little girl is still there. I imagine her climbing onto her horse and soaring high and free, leaving the pain far behind her . . . a distant memory.

A NOTE FROM MOMMY

Dearest Jade,

There is so much I want to say to you — so many things I would have handled differently in life and so many things that just happened that I could not control. But the one thing I can say is that I truly love you more than life itself. You are the most wonderful thing I have ever done in my life and the one thing I would never question or change. Holding you in my arms brought new meaning to the word "Love," and that love and admiration for you continue to grow. I wanted to give you the most glorious life, and for a time, I felt that I did — but I have also learned from you, that we look at life differently. When you were only three years old, I remember my own mother saying to me, "Ava, she is smarter than you and stronger than you — It is going to be some ride!" And well, my beautiful daughter — it has been! You are gorgeous and smart and talented and courageous — and I think I got my courage from you, rather than the other way around. You have taught me so much and you continue to amaze me when we talk. I am beyond aware that my illness and heart transplant changed both of us forever, and for that, I am sorry. I never wanted things to be so hard for you and I never wanted to be the thing that held you back in your life. I am so proud of how you have always continued to move through life, accepting and conquering challenges and chasing your dreams. Watching you jump your pony for the first time gave me chills and the look on your little face after winning is emblazoned in my memory. Priceless. You were fearless and I hope — I want — you to be fearless again in your life. Maybe you are. I know only that you are the reason I lived. I did see the Light and I wanted to go to it. I wanted to die, because it was easy and beautiful and painless. But there you were on the other side with your dirty horse hair — pulling me back. I cannot explain the sense of needing to come back to you, but God let me come. You were only eleven and you had to be so brave. You dug deep into your soul and you survived and thrived. You are my everything, and I know the path I have chosen has not been easy. Someone gave me a life back and I made a promise that if I could come back and have the honor of being your Mom, I would spend the rest of my life giving back. I know I have kept my promise with Ava's Heart and the countless families that I — we — have helped. Without you, there would have been no me. I hope that somewhere inside of you, you are proud of me as well, for continuing to see through all of my promises and following my beautiful new heart. The people we have helped have all been because of you.

When I close my eyes, I can hear your voice singing, and I remember the first time I heard that voice at a musical theater. I asked the other moms, "Who is that singing?" And they said, "That's Jade!" You always continue to surprise me and I am in awe of your talent and strength. I am glad we go through normal mother and daughter turmoil sometimes because it gives me hope that you are okay.

Your time is now, Baby Girl. Go fly high and create those big dreams of yours. I am fine. Be free and unafraid. Know that you have not only saved my life, but the lives of so many other people — just because you are you. We both know we cannot change what happened to us, but we can change how we deal with all of it. Not a day goes by that you are not inside of me. Mommy and Jade — I love who we are, who we have been, and who we are about to become.

Mommy

Jade Kaufman

The Reason Why Ava Lived

Daughter, Friend, Protector

Equestrian, Actress, Singer

Extraordinary Human Being

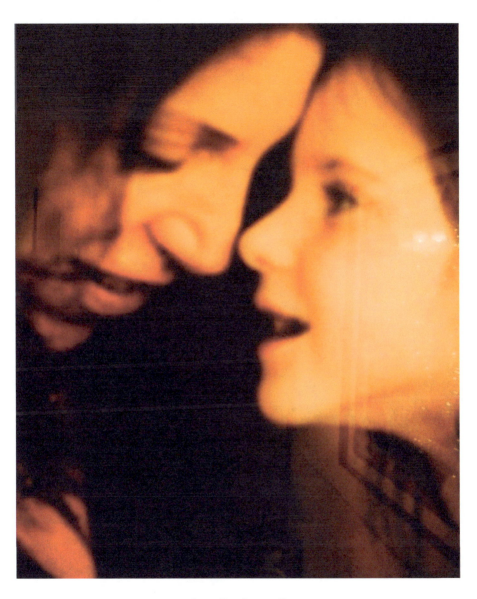

Ava and Jade shared a secret

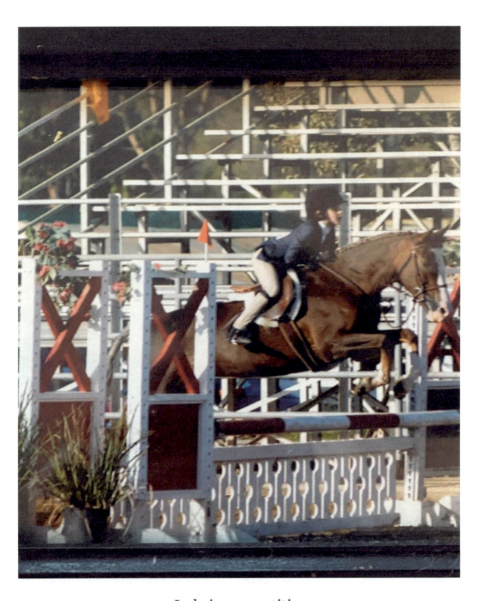

Jade in competition

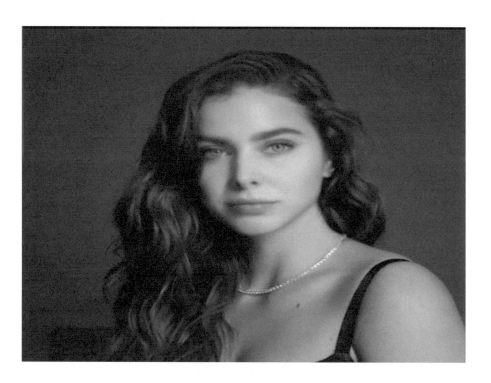

Jade Kaufman – The reason Ava lived

CHAPTER THIRTY-FIVE
AVA'S HEART - BUILDING AN EVER-EVOLVING COMMUNITY

AVA AND ME

Ava:

For some of the people we have written about in this book, it feels like things will never be okay again. And for others, they dedicate their lives to making sure things are always on a better road.

There is a moment when we can quiet our minds and rid our thoughts of what we think we should be doing or who we think we should be. In that quiet space, we can exhale our fears and sadness. We know that time marches on, without hesitation and without bias for those left behind. This too shall pass, as will each and every one of us.

With all of that being said, I needed to take a long, hard look at where I have come from in my life and think about where I am going and why. I realize not everyone gets to have as many chances at life as I have so generously been given. When people say "everything happens for a reason," I can honestly say that, like karma, that is not entirely true. There may not be a reason for why I lived while others did not, but I can *make* a reason. I can look back at how I have conducted myself throughout my life and assess if that will help me in my current endeavors or not. Perseverance can go a long way, but if I can't follow at least some of the rules and restrictions, I understand now, on the eve of my 71st birthday, that while *some* rules are made to be broken, others are made so that things can work out. I made a promise to God to spend the rest of my life being a great Mom and helping people who are in need in the transplant community. I understand a lot now, not only because I had my own heart transplant but because of the lack of community and understanding devoted to my recovery. My Uncle Saul wanted me to move to Florida and live with Claire after my transplant. With his suggestion, which was supported by my family, there were two things that were very clear to me. First, my family proposed that I live somewhere where there was no transplant center, and that should anything go wrong with my precious new heart, which was a most beautiful gift, there would be nowhere for me to go for help. This was not a family who furiously researched what I was going through and how they could help me recover and move forward with my life. And that brings me to my second point. The realization that they wanted me to learn some lesson that they thought I had clearly missed and now it was time for me to quietly accept some fate I had invited into my life. But that was what I learned. Each person who has gone through a transplant lives with a new reality — a new life — and recovery cannot happen if we go quietly away. The idea was not to be silenced. It was to speak more loudly and to scream until people would listen. We all need help one way or another and to have the understanding to reach out and be there for each other — to be a part of a community for the benefit of someone we may not know makes us better as human beings.

Coming to terms with myself has been the single most difficult part of this whole process. I have spent my entire life fighting to do what I wanted: a more exciting life — a crazy handsome husband or a lover unmatched by any other one before. But my vision has always been greater than my current position. I could always see where a company could go, but I didn't always know how to get there. With Ava's Heart, I see that has not changed. I know where the transplant community *needs* to be to help heal the patients, but my passion alone cannot get us there. I have met and written about some truly extraordinary people in this book. We have tried to put a human story into every chapter because not one single one of us ever thought we would be here today, but the other thing we have in common is that we pushed and pushed to recover and we find ourselves talking about the people we have met along the way. We are a community now, but that has not always been the case. There is a story behind every life gained and every life lost. Transplant recipients were previously not "allowed" to contact the donor families. We are not perfect. There will not always be a right answer in the transplant community. Not all donor families want to meet the recipients of their loved ones' organs. Doctors sometimes say that families look for the transference between the donors and their recipients. But like everything else since the history of the world began, nothing is perfect. We sometimes have moments where we feel like we touched perfection, but that doesn't ever last. And maybe that's the secret — understanding that this is a process. It will not always work out how we think it should, but then there's a new challenge and we have to switch gears to make things work. I would love to meet my donor family one day, just to let them know that I have worked every single day to honor my precious gift. But I understand with equal measure and without judgement that they are not ready for that.

Because nothing is perfect.

I can see a community where there are homes in every transplant-available city, where families can live and recover from their transplants. Every time I see an empty building, I imagine the number of people we could help, and there could be places for people to talk about their experiences in a group. Every story in this book has made me weep for different reasons. And if I had never had my transplant, I would never have met this extraordinary group of people. I live in Los Angeles, where two of the largest transplant centers in the world are located. Families *need* what I do. I am one person with one house. I have to turn people away every day. Yes, people die waiting for an organ because there are not enough donors. But people also die because without post-transplant housing, they cannot even get listed. They don't die waiting on a list — they can't even get *on* the list. Both of these issues are fixable.

K.B. Hill:

I find myself at a crossroads now. As I moved through the writing of this extraordinary book, I listened to people carefully and pulled everything I could from their words — their looks — the sounds of their voices, sometimes individual but always in unison for the patients. I found it astounding how perfectly, how uniquely qualified the professionals all are for their jobs. It's amazing to know that if you ever needed them, there are people out there who believe in helping you so wholeheartedly, with absolute and unabashed purity, you would be in the hands of angels. My friend Ava is one of those people. Things have come full circle for me, because as we approach Ava's 71st birthday (her 12th birthday with her Shark Heart), I remember the day she woke up and thought I was an angel standing at the end of her bed. But it is, in fact, the other way around. Every person I wrote about broke my heart, gave me hope, lifted me up, while I sobbed, trying to tell their stories to the very best of my ability. I don't know that there was a single chapter I wrote where I didn't cry. Knowing what these people have lived with, endured, lost — well it gives you more perspective on your own life. I always look for that common thread in my writing. Sometimes, when working on a thriller, I jump back and forth between times and characters until they all come together, and magically, that has happened with Shark Heart.

Ava is the common thread. The community that she has amassed is the purpose. Being sick is scary, and I believe that after a devastating year of Covid-19, we can all attest to that. One of the people I interviewed for this book had called Ava while I was with her. I heard her on the phone, trying to get through her brother's story. Even though the call was private, I heard her and I felt her pain. By the time the call was done, I felt like I was choking. When Ava asked me to interview her, I, of course, agreed. But it was so tough. Listening to her, I imagined the brother she spoke of, so alive, riding his bicycle through the streets of Los Angeles, helping the homeless when he could. I imagined a slender young man on a bicycle, riding as fast as he could. I imagined a thick mop of dark hair, under which deep, warm brown eyes took in the world around him, as he calculated who he could help next. I think about him parking his bicycle outside of the church, where he would visit his friend, the priest, and talk about life and people. I wonder, how did this young man have such a firm and understanding grasp on humanity? I imagine that when he asked his mother about reincarnation, and told her he wanted to come back as a bird, I know why. I know that being able to fly would have given him a broader picture of the world, soaring high and fast above the streets where he once rode his bicycle . . .

I'm crying again.

He became a part of Ava's community through his sister. Each of the people I interviewed on Ava's behalf is not only a part of her own journey, but they have made great contributions to their own communities. Ava's Heart is such an important part of that and I don't think the full meaning of that hit me until I spoke with the professionals. There is a need that is hidden in organ transplantation. It is true that people die waiting for a match, but it is also true that people die because they can't even get listed if they don't have post-operative housing available to them. The three rooms Ava can provide at her house don't come close to where she needs to be for her foundation to be a fully operative part of the community. The small donation she receives to help donor families bury their loved ones doesn't cover everyone. Sometimes, she drops her head and has to say no. Ava is one small woman — tiny, actually. She uses her unbreakable shark heart to gather the community, fight for people she has never met, and to give them a moment of reprieve at the worst time of their lives. She does it because she made a promise to God and because she knows how it feels — because Jenna Rush, a nurse — told her it's what people need and what is not available is this messy, complicated procedure. Someone figured out how to transplant an organ — to remove a heart, or a lung or a kidney — and replace it with a new one — doctors and nurses got on board, because it's what they do. They help people — they save lives — they spend years in school, and then re-educate themselves every time something new and miraculous is discovered — and they learn how it works — so they can save even more people. Ava is not a doctor, but she is a patient. There was a great need and she is using every fiber of her being to fill that need. She is building a community and she listens to hundreds of stories like the handful of the stories in this book. Her heart must be strong.

Her heart must be strong.

Each of these people goes out into the world every day, looking to make a difference in their own lives and the lives of those they come in contact with, allowing the community to continue to grow. In other parts of the country, there are entire apartment complexes dedicated to what Ava does, but that doesn't exist here. So she is pushing to make it happen. The doctor and nurses, patients and patient advocates, and the families and friends of everyone involved understand there are pieces missing from a puzzle, but they are trying to find them and get them in place, so that each person who becomes a part of the transplant family is able to heal fully and completely, and so that donor families are never left unable to bury their loved ones.

Ava's community is not made up of doctors who became doctors because they wanted to get a good paycheque. They are people who understand humanity on a molecular level. They are people who believe that they can travel around the world and get other countries to understand the altruistic need of making every single person a donor. They are the people who whispered to her that someone needed her help — just so they could get listed to get their life-saving organ transplant. They are people who receive a second chance at life, and use it to try to help others understand the journey, should they or anyone they love ever need to become a part of their own transplant journey. And they are families who tell stories of their loved ones, who gave the ultimate gift and are finding ways to create hope again. They are Ava's own friends — some old and some new, who had lifted her up and supported her when it all became too much — when the stories and phone calls from people she could not help made her feel like her tears for them would drown her.

And they are all connected to each other — through Ava's new heart.

I have always believed one hundred percent in the things that we cannot see as being the stories that bind us together. We cannot *see* love, but we can experience it — feel it, give it, take it away, cherish it and let it go. We cannot see mythical creatures, but they have transcended time and borders of countries, cultures and even religions — and yet we all have versions of those same creatures. We cannot account for everything the human brain can imagine or achieve, but we can find our place in a world that may be heavily divided by simply helping people who are in need heal. We cannot see mental illness, but it is everywhere. We cannot see a person's quiet pain, but we can listen to them and find ways to make their pain better. The answers are all out there — if we can learn to listen to others and take them in and find common ground. There were people in this book who think very differently than I do about many things. But I focused on what we have in common. Being a mother, for instance.

That's what brought Ava back. Being a mother.

I didn't want to bring the year 2020 into this story, because I wanted it to be timeless so that many years from now, if someone were to read it, they would find a way to make their own community better or stronger — to find understanding where perhaps there had not previously been before. But in this past year, the stories of the doctors and nurses who held iPads for loved ones to say goodbye to their family and friends who were taken because of Covid — who held them in their last moments of life — spoke volumes to me about the power and humanity expressed by these people every single day. They became a part of another human's life as they drew their last breath, and the next day, they did it again . . . and again. But those are the stories that Ava hears every day. She reaches out to as many as she can. She helps every person she can — but like the people who died before the iPad was turned on, or before the nurse could get to the room, a few lives slipped away. Those were the lives of any of us — of all of us, because *"there, but for the Grace of God, go I."*

Ava, you are an angel. And I have met quite a few while writing this book. I am humbled by your friendship.

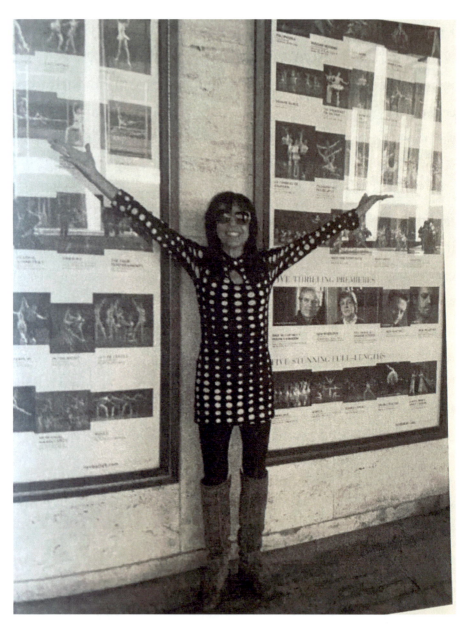

Ava Babbin Kaufman – Survivor, Activist, Mother and Friend

A dream of a swimming shark is to remind you that you are powerful

Made in United States
Troutdale, OR
12/02/2024

25651135R00148